# Tibetan Medicine :
# Theory and Practice

Indian Medicinal Science Series No.-54

# Tibetan Medicine : Theory and Practice

## Vaidya Bhagwan Dash

Sri Satguru Publications

*A Division of*

Indian Books Centre

Delhi, India

*Published by:*
**Sri Satguru Publications**
Indological and Oriental Publishers
*A Division of*
**Indian Books Centre**
40/5, Shakti Nagar,
Delhi-110007
(INDIA)

First Edition: Delhi, 1997

ISBN 81-7030-519-5

Printed in India

Published by Sunil Gupta for Sri Satguru Publications, a division of Indian Books Centre, 40/5, Shakti Nagar, Delhi and Printed at Mehra Offset Press, Delhi.

# Preface

To overcome the galloping incidence of obstinate and often incurable diseases, both physical and mental, to arrest the growing disharmony in the society, and to remedy the frustration among the youth because of disturbed family life, an alternative way of living and an alternative system of health care are being considered seriously all over the world. Tibet, the land of mysteries and mystics which remained closed to the outside world for a long time in the past, and which has opened up now, is a vast store house of knowledge in this direction. Unnoticed, and therefore, unacknowledged, this magnificient land of so far unpolluted or less polluted environment, vibrates with energy to rejuvenate the present day ailing humanity.

The traditional medicine of Tibet, still popular among the local inhabitants and those of the border regions of the neighbouring countries, is a conglomeration of science, art, philosophy and religion, one closely depending upon the other. It has its own concepts of composition of the universe and body, physiology, pharmacology and pathology. It has its unique way of diagnosing diseases and treating them. The physician is considered to be an epitome of physical, mental and spiritual virtues.

Several books and xylographs on Tibetan medicine are available in Tibetan. More recently, some useful books are also published in English and other foreign languages. In the present work an effort has been made to give an exposition of important aspects of this health science in brief. The efforts of the author will be well rewarded if it proves to be useful to students, physicians and research workers in this unique field.

**Vaidya Bhagwan Dash**

# Contents

# Introduction

Man has eternally endeavoured to keep himself free from three types of miseries, viz., those arising out of one's own physique, those caused by environmental factors including harmful microbes surrounding him, and those caused by supernatural bodies including evil spirits. Health is not merely freedom from physical ailments. To be really healthy, a person should be mentally happy, socially secured and spiritually elevated with his senses functioning perfectly till his death, in addition to freedom from these physical ailments.

Since time immemorial, different ethical and social rules were stipulated to prevent mental aberrations and to maintain social harmony. Different religious doctrines were propagated with philosophical background to help people to achieve spiritual enlightenment. Different diet, drinks and drugs were repeatedly experimented upon and used to prevent and cure these ailments, and to preserve and promote positive health. Some of these drugs, diet and drinks were used empirically as found in the folk-medicines of different countries. But in the ancient cradles of civilization, the use of these drugs, etc.; were rationalised with scientific concepts and explanations. Tibetan medicine is one such rational and scientific system for the upkeep of the health of the humanity where science, art, philosophy, ethics and religion are interwoven into one fabric.

Modern medical science, of late has made considerable progress in various fields. The era of specialization and the tendency to see the man as a physico-chemical entity of many separate parts is giving place to a new genre of biological and holistic thinking. The new school of thought is directed towards the concept of the man as a whole person with his physical, emotional, social and spiritual aspects inseparably unified in one living individual. The place of man as an organic part of the biological and cosmic universe subject to all the immutable and irrevocable laws of nature is being increasingly recognised.

In spite of these profound changes taking place in medical thought, today's conventional drug approach of modern medicine is unable to solve the catastrophic increase in such diseases as AIDS, cancer, cardio-vascular disorders, diabetes, asthma, arthritis, liver disorders and so forth. Many of these diseases are declared as 'incurable'. People are made to believe that pain-killers, antibiotics and steroids which give temporary relief, and whose continued use has serious toxic effects are the only way out. The net result of this criminal negligence has left thousands of crippled and unproductive men, women and children all over the world.

The other side of the story is that the traditional medicine of Tibet and such other countries do have successful treatment for these so called "incurable diseases".

## Unique Features of Tibetan Medicine

Prior to the arrival of Buddhism (*chos*), a form of Samanism (*bon*) was in practice in Tibet. The present day traditional medicine of Tibet is a fine conglomeration of the folk-tradition earlier practised by *bon-pas*, and the rational scientific stream which arrived there along with Buddhism. Following are the unique features of the present day traditional medicine of Tibet :

## (1) **Holistic Approach**

A disease may appear in a particular part of the body. Apart from the organ in which the disease is manifested, several other organs or tissues of the body are affected to cause the disease. Each disease has a site of origin, and the path of circulation for the morbid material to be transported from the site of origin to the site of manifestation of the disease. Therefore, while diagnosing and treating a disease the body as a whole is taken into account, and not only the affected organ or part of the body. Since during treatment the morbid material from the whole body is taken out, the disease is not just suppressed but completely rooted out.

## (2) **Psycho-somatic Concept**

For the causation of a disease, both the physical and mental factors are involved. Anger, passion and illusion (ignorance) may constitute the causative factors of the physical diseases. Similarly, physical factors like bad food and regimens may cause mental disorders. Because of this psycho-somatic concept of the disease, the practitioners of Traditional Tibetan Medicine prescribe many regimens and conducts including religious practices, along with drugs, diet and drinks while treating a patient.

## (3) **Field is More Important Than Seed**

Invading and harmful microbes are considered to be the causative factors of several diseases. But these microbes are treated only as secondary causative factors, the primary factors being the disturbance in the equilibrium of *nad* or *ñes-pa*-s (three factors which control the body physiology), *lus-zuṅ*-s (seven categories of tissue elements) and *dri-ma*-s (waste products of digestion and metabolism). If the field or soil is barren, the seed howsoever potent it may be, when sown, will not germinate. Similarly, when there is harmony among *ñes-pa*-s etc., then the invading microbe howsoever virulant it may be will not be able to multiply and grow in the body to cause a disease. The traditional physician of Tibet, therefore prescribes drugs, diet, drinks, regimens and religious practices to maintain this equilibrium or homeostasis, and not to kill these invading organisms.

## (4) No Side Toxic Effects But Side Benefits

Invading microbes are certainly more powerful than the body cells. Any medicine which is given to destroy the invading microbes is certainly more powerful, and naturally it produces harmful effects on the body cells. These harmful effects are manifested in the form of side-toxic reactions. Left to themselves the body cells have the inherent power to attack and destroy these invading organisms which may of course take some time. Use of antibiotics to destroy these microbes do not allow that opportunity to body cells to develop immunity or resistance power. Thus, they suffer from the attacks by these microbes again and again. Repeated use of these antibiotics also makes these microbes drug-resistant. On the other hand, the physicians of Tibetan medicine prescribe drugs, diet and regimens, which while bringing about the equilibrium of *ñes-pa*-s etc., promote the immunity of the body against these invading organisms by which they succumb to their inevitable death. This increased immunity prevents further attacks by the microbes. Restoration of the equilibrium among the functional and structural units makes the body clean and strong. Thus, instead of side-toxic reactions, drugs of Tibetan medicine produce several side benefits.

## (5) Every Medicine is a Tonic

Since the drugs of Tibetan medicine do not aim at killing the invading microbes but primarily aim at maintaining equilibrium among the functional and structural units in the body, all of them work as tonics. These recipes are equally useful for both the patients and healthy persons. In the former, these recipes cure the diseases, and in the latter, they promote the immunitary system, and thus work as tonics. Even, otherwise toxic ingredients like aconite, mercury, sulphur and arsenic work as tonics as these are carefully detoxicated and made homologous before being included in recipes.

## (6) Non-toxic Nature of Medicines

Drugs of modern medicine including the synthetic chemicals are marketed for therapeutic use after testing them for acute toxicity, sub-acute toxicity, chronic toxicity and terratogenic effects. In spite of this scientific scrutiny, some of these are banned later because of their harmful effects on the body. Thus, marketing a drug after scientifically establishing its therapeutic utility and non-toxic nature, and later banning it for its inefficacy and toxicity has become so common that a drug imported for use in one country stands banned in the country of its origin before it reaches its destination. On the other hand, drugs of Tibetan medicine are in use for thousands of years and they have maintained their therapeutic efficacy and non-toxic nature even till today.

## (7) Use of Natural Ingredients

Raw drugs used in Tibetan medicine are natural ones. Synthetic drugs or isolated fractions like alkaloids and glucosides are not used in this traditional system. In these raw drugs, naturally alkaloids, etc., are present. Use of these active principles alone, in addition to curing diseases, may produce adverse effects. In the same plant, there are other fractions which counteract the harmful effects of these so called active principles. In any way, in Tibetan medicine, a plant is never used for its alkaloid content etc. It is selected on the basis of its *ro*'(taste), etc., which will be discussed in detail at a later stage.

## (8) Simple Manufacturing Processes and Socialistic Approach

Preparing medicines from the raw ingredients does not involve any sophisticated and high technology. The traditional physicians themselves manufacture their medicines for their patients. For convenience, at times, these medicines are manufactured by centralised organisations which also does not involve any high technology. The ingredients are processed only to make them free from any untoward effect, and to make the final products delicious, easily digestible, assimilable, therapeutically more potent and preservable.

Raw ingredients are collected by the physicians with the assistance of local people from natural sources. Some of these ingredients are also cultivated. People who assist in the collection of these herbs, etc., from the forests and fields, those who cultivate them, and semi-skilled workers who assist in the manufacture of final products share the profit and earn their livelihood.

## (9) Cheapness of Medicines

Since local flora and fauna are mostly used in the manufacture of these medicines, and the use of sophisticated equipments and technology is not involved, these medicines are generally very cheap and people of low economic status can easily afford. Medicines containing costly gems, etc., are no doubt, a little expensive. But such medicines are generally used for the treatment of obstinate and otherwise incurable diseases. Thus in ultimate analysis even such costly drugs become economical.

## (10) Environmental Protection

Drugs use in Tibetan medicine are, for the most part collected from the forests and fields. Their preservation, protection and development are, therefore, of great interest to the traditional physicians of Tibet. No big factories, no air pollution and no pollution of river water are, therefore, the basic requirements of Tibetan medicine.

## (11) Emphasis on Positive Health

Treatment of disease after it is manifested is, no doubt, undertaken by the traditional physicians of Tibet. But the main objective of Tibetan medicine is to prevent the occurrence of diseases, and to preserve as well as promote positive health. For this purpose, several regimens and conducts for different parts of the day and night, and for different seasons are described in Tibetan medical classics and prescribed by the Tibetan physicians.

## (12) Emphasis on Diet

For the maintenance of positive health, and for the prevention as well as cure of diseases, Tibetan traditional medicine lays considerable emphasis on diet and drinks. With proper diet, the disease get cured without needing much of medicines and without proper diet the disease does not get cured in spite of the best of medicines. Therefore, while treating a patient, along with medicines, the physician invariably prescribes what type of food to be taken and which are to be avoided.

## (13) Interdependability of Microcosm and Macrocosm

According to Tibetan medicine, the individual is a microcosm, and it is an exact replica of the macrocosm or the universe. Every phenomenon of the universe takes place in the individual, and every activity of the individual affects the universe. Here comes the role of *mantras* or religious incantations through the practice of which, a person can purify himself, and control the environment.

## (14) Belief in Karma

Buddhism believes in the existence of the past life and life after death. Actions of the past life are partially consumed in that life itself, and some of the results of the actions of the past life called *karma* are carried forward to the present life to produce obstinate and incurable diseases. When such diseases are manifested, the patient does not draw any significant benefit from ordinary modes of treatment. Special therapeutic measures including religious rituals are prescribed for the treatment of such diseases.

## (15) Unification of Science, Philosophy and Religion

Tibetan traditional medicine is a conglomeration of science, philosophy and religion. Without one the other two are incomplete. For a person to be happy and healthy, practice of religious prescriptions is considered essential. Here, religion does not refer to Buddhism alone. One should follow the religion of his own faith and lead a religious life.

This is emphasised both for the physician and the patient equally.

## Specialised Branches of Tibetan Medicine

The traditional medicine of Tibet has eight specialised branches as follows :

(1) *Lus* or the description of the body including embryology, anatomy, physiology, pathology, pharmacology and diagnosis as well as treatment of diseases affecting the body in general;

(2) *Byis-pa* or management of the specific requirements of the infant after delivery, and treatment of the diseases specially occurring in the child;

(3) *Mo-nad* or the management of ailments occurring specially in mothers including gynaecology;

(4) *Gdon* or the description of the evil spirits and diagnosis as well as treatment of ailments caused by them;

(5) *Mtson* or the description of surgical ailments and their management;

(6) *Dug* or the description of various categories of poisons, and diagnosis as well as treatment of toxicological ailments;

(7) *Rgyas* or geriatrics including description of rejuvenation therapies for the prevention as well as cure of geriatric ailments; and

(8) *Ro-tsa* or the description of fertility, reproductivity including the treatment of impotency and sterility through aphrodisiac therapies.

Due to temporal vicissitude, some of these specialised branches are less practised. But Tibetan medical classics are replete with the description of these specialised branches.

# 1

# Historical Background

History of Tibetan Medicine, and its origin are shrouded with myths, legends, anecdotes and facts like those of other countries and cultures. The earliest inhabitants of Tibet, "the Land of Snow" perhaps practised a form of Shamanism which was prevalent in the whole of Northern Asia, and it was known as 'Bon'. The followers of this tradition, called Bon-pas had a rich tradition of medicine as the recently (in 1972) published four works composed by Khyuṅ-sprul 'Jigs-med Nam-kha'i Rdo-rje indicate.

During the reign of the king Sroṅ-btsan sgam-po (c. 620-650) Buddhism was introduced in Tibet which highly influenced the culture and tradition of Tibetans. It was called 'Chos'. The King sent a band of Tibetan intellectuals headed by his Finance Minister named Tho-mi Saṃbhota to India for preparing a script for Tibetan language, and to study Buddhist scriptures in the land of its origin. These scholars acquired the knowledge of various arts and sciences, in addition to Buddhist scriptures prevalent in India at that time. They thereafter, translated these scriptures into Tibetan language. These scriptures, along with those composed later, were compiled into Bka'-'gyur (Kanjur) and Bstan-'gyur (Tanjur) at a subsequent period.

The King had two wives, one from China and the other from Nepal. The Chinese princess brought along with her, a medical text entitled Sman-dpyad Chen-mo from China which was later translated into Tibetan by Ha-shaṅ Mahādeva and Dharma-kośa.

The King also invited doctors from India, China and Persia for the translation of the medical texts of their own countries. After the translation, they jointly prepared a medical text entitled *Mi 'Jigs-pa'i Mtson-cha* comprising seven chapters, and presented it to the King.

In the beginning of eighth century, Khri-lde Gtsug-btan became the King of Tibet, and Bran-ti was his court physician. Many medical texts on the basis of his instructions were composed later by his disciples.

Later, Mes-'ag-tsoms (fl. 710 A.D.) became the King of Tibet, and his son married to a Chinese princess who brought along with her medical and astrological texts from China and these were translated into Tibetan. During this period, Bi-byi or Campasila translated and composed several medical texts, and his sons became reputed physicians of Tibet. He was appointed as the Court physician. During this period, in order to regulate medical practice and to honour the Medical profession, the King promulgated rules (six for beneficiaries and one for the physician) as follows :

(1)  The court physician should on all occasions be offered a seat of honour;
(2)  He should have the best of cushions to seat;
(3)  He should be offered the best food;
(4)  He should be taken and sent back on horse back;
(5)  Gratitude to him should always be remembered; and
(6)  He should be paid in gold.

The physician should treat his patients with love and compassion and should treat them as his own sons and daughters. He should not demand or take any food or drink in the house of the patient.

During the time between the King Mes-'ag-tshoms (fl. 710 A.D.) and coronation of the King Khri-sron lde-btsan (754 A.D.) many medical texts were translated into Tibetan.

During the reign of the King Khri-sroṅ lde-btsan (754-780 A.D.) two Indian saints, namely Śānta-rakṣita and Padma-sambhava came to Tibet to preach Buddhism. Padma-sambhava was also a physician, and he wrote a book entitled *Bdud-rtsi Sñiṅ-po*.

Padma-sambhava's disciple Vairocana came to India, and learnt medicine from twenty five scholar physicians. From Candra-nandana, he learnt *Amṛta-hṛdaya-aṣṭāṅga-guhyopadeśa-tantra* and translated it into Tibetan which is popularly known as *Rgyud-bźi*. The translated work was presented to the King when his teacher Padma-sambhava, and Gyu-thog Yon-tan Mgon-po were present.

The King Khri-sroṅ lde-btsan invited several foreign physicians to Tibet from India, Kashmir, China, Persia, Guge, Dol-po and Nepal to translate the medical texts of their respective countries into Tibetan. Apart from this translation work, they also trained nine intelligent Tibetan boys in Medicine. These nine physicians, thereafter were appointed as court-physicians of the King. One of these physicians was Gyu-thog Yon-tan Mgon-po (the Senior) who later become the most reputed physicians of Tibet.

During this period, the Senior Gyu-thog-pa visited India three times for further study of medicine, and wrote several masterly medical works. In his biography, details of his visits to different parts of India, and his training in medicine are described.

The Chief physician of the court of the King Khri-sroṅ lde-btsan was a Chinese doctor who composed a medical text on his way from China to Tibet which was presented to the King. He cured the King's illness for which he was awarded land and other facilities, and made to settle in Tibet.

During the reign of the later King Glan-dar-ma, Buddhism received a set back, and the religious institutions were destroyed. In spite of it, the medical tradition of Tibet, adopted earlier, continued uninterrupted.

During the reign of the King Lha-bla-ma Ye-ses-'od, in the later half of tenth century, the Indian Pandit Dharma-śrī-varman, Sñe-bo lo-tsa-ba Dbyig-gi Rin-chen and others translated the famous auto-commentary (*Vaidūryaka-bhāṣya*) on Vāgbhaṭa's work called *Yan-lag-Brgyad-pa'i Sñiṅ-po Bsdus-pa.*

During this period, the Great translator Rin-chen Bzaṅ-po (958 -1055 A.D.) went to India, and stayed there for four years to learn Buddhist scriptures and Medicine. From a Kashmiri physician called Janārdana, he learnt *Yan-lag Brgyad-pa'i Sñiṅ-po Bsdus-pa (Aṣṭāṅga-hṛdaya-saṃhitā)* and its famous commentary *Padārtha-candrikā* by Candra-nandana. He translated these texts into Tibetan. His successors and disciples wrote commentaries on *Rgyud-bźi* and several other medical texts. Some of his successors went to India, and learnt Medicine from Ṛṣi Candrāvi (Candrasila). After return to Tibet, they composed several works on Medicine.

In the eleventh century, the Junior Gyu-thog Yon-tan Mgon-po (who belonged to the religious tradition of the Senior Gyu-thog-pa described earlier) visited India and Śrīlaṅkā six times to study Medicine. He wrote twenty books on Medicine.

During the 14th century, there were two famous doctors in Tibet, namely Byaṅs-pa and Zur-mkhar-pa. Byaṅs-pa became very famous during the reign of the Second Dalai Lama (1391-1475 A.D.). He wrote many original medical texts, and commentaries on *Rgyud-bźi*. His successors, similarly composed several works on Medicine and commentary on the whole of *Rgyud-bźi*. This tradition was popularly known as *Byaṅ-lugs*. The other famous doctor Zur-mkhar-pa also wrote a commentary on *Rgyud-bźi* and the tradition thus created was called *Zur-lugs*.

After this period, Buddhism became very popular in Mongolia and Lama Physicians of Tibet were appointed as Court physicians there.

The Fifth Dalai Lama (1617-1682 A.D.) established a Medical School at Dga' ldan Pho-braṅ in 'Bras-spun Monastery. During his time, an organised Medical school was established at Lcags-po-ri which is still continuing its training and treatment programmes.

After the death of the fifth Dalai Lama, the succeeding regent Sde-srid Saṅs-rgyas Rgya-mtsho (1653 - 1705 A.D.) wrote a commentary on *Rgyud-bźi* called *Bai du rya Sṅon-po*. Besides, he wrote several works on Medicine.

During the reign of the thirteenth Dalai Lama (1895 - 1933 A.D.) a new college of Medicine and Astrology called *Sman-rtsi-khaṅ* was established in Lhasa near Gtsug-la-khaṅ. This college was organised and headed by a reputed Tibetan physician Mkhyen-rab Nor-bu (1882-1962 A.D.). This college is still continuing to impart training and treatment.

The 14th Dalai Lama (b. 1935 A.D.– ), because of political turmoil in Tibet, came to India, and established his head-quarters at Dharmashala in 1959 A.D. A Medical School was established by His Holiness at Dharmashala in 1961 to provide medical aid for migrated Tibetans and the local Indian population. This Medical school was organised by His Holiness's personal physician Ye-se Don-den (b. 1927 A.D.– ). Apart from the training centre, this Institution is equipped with an Out Patient Department, Hospital, Pharmacy and Library. This Institution has become so popular that patients from far of regions of India and also from abroad are coming there for medical help. Foreign doctors are also provided here facilities for training in Tibetan Medicine. The graduates of this college are now providing medical help to suffering humanity in different centres in India and abroad.

## 2

## Rgyud-bźi : The Celebrated Text of Tibetan Medicine

Eventhough number of foreign doctors were invited to Tibet, several foreign medical works were got translated into Tibetan, and several foreign physicians were appointed as court physicians during different periods of the history of Tibet of which recorded evidence is still available in Tibetan, it is only some of the Indian Ayurvedic texts that were incorporated into the Tibetan scriptures, and the noncanonical medical text which reigned supreme in the life and culture of Tibetans is *Rgyud-bźi*. It is this *Rgyud-bźi* which is popularly followed for training of physicians in Tibet, Bhutan and Mongolia, and the traditional physicians of these countries follow the instructions provided in this text for the preservation and promotion of positive health of their people, and prevention as well as cure of the diseases of their patients.

The original text of *Rgyud-bźi* was composed in Sanskrit, and its original title was *Amṛta-hṛdaya-aṣṭāṅga-guhyopadeśa-tantra*. It was later translated into Tibetan, and the Tibetan title coined for this translated work is *Bdud-rtsi Sñiṅ-po Yan-lag-brgyad-pa Gsaṅ-ba Man-ṅag-gi Rgyud*. Since this work is divided into four different treatises, it is popularly known as *Rgyud* (treatises) - *bźi* (four) or the "Compendium of Four Treatises".

The name of the original author does not appear in any part of the book. The writer perhaps intentionally omitted it because of his humbleness and modesty. Since the work was composed under the instructions of Lord Buddha, incorporating the name of human-author to this divine work was perhaps considered inappropriate.

According to historical tradition as enshrined in zur-lugs or the school of Zur-mkhar Mnam-nis Rdo-rje, and quoted by the famous commentator Sde-srid Saṅs-rgyas Rgya-mtsho in pp 358-359 of his *khog-'bugs* (Pub.: T.Y. Gangpa, Leh, 1970), it was Jīvaka or Kumāra Jīvaka (Tib.: Tsho-byed Gźon-nu) who was the first recipient of this divine knowledge from Lord Buddha. It was this Kumāra Jīvaka who because of his profound knowledge in medicine was thrice crowned as the King of physicians by Lord Buddha Himself.

As has been mentioned before, Vairocana (also written as Bairocana), during the reign of the King Khri-sroṅ lde-btsan (754-780 A.D.) went to India at the instructions of his teacher Padma-sambhava, and learnt this text from Candra-nandana who was the descendant of Vāgbhaṭa. After learning it, he translated the text into Tibetan, and presented it to the King in the presence of his teacher Padma-sambhava and the reputed physician of that time Gyu-thog Yon-tan Mgon-pa. Padma-sambhava did not think that time to be appropriate for the Tibetans to accept and adopt this work. Therefore, on his advice, this translated text was kept hidden as *gter-ma* in one of the pillars of the central hall of the upper shrine of Sam-ye (Bsam-yas) monastery near Lhasa. As predicted by the teacher this work was taken out of the pillar in 1038 A.D. by Gter-ston Gra-pa Mṅon-śes and widely propagated in Tibet.

During this period (8th cent. A.D.), G'yu-thog Yon-tan Mgon-pa (the elder or senior) visited India three times. He was earlier acquainted with Vairocana's translation of *Rgyud-bźi*, and revised it with the help of the physicians of India. His

descendant in the line of succession G'yu-thog Yon-tan
Mgon-pa, the Junior, visited India for six times in 11th cent.
A.D. Apart from writing several original medical texts, he
also revised *Rgyud-bźi* with his updated knowledge.

In 13th cent. A.D. the sovereignty of Tibet was
recognised by Mongolian rulers, and Lama Doctors were
appointed as Court physicians of Mongolia. During this
period, *Rgyud-bźi* was translated into Mongolian (from
Tibetan), and became popular in that country. Several
commentaries were written on this work, and several medical
texts in Mongolian were composed on the basis of this
*Rgyud-bźi*.

In the fourteenth century, the then two reputed Tibetan
doctors, namely, Byaṅs-pa and Zur-mkhar-pa wrote two
different commentaries which were conceptually different.
This gave rise to two schools of thought in the field of
medicine, viz., *Byaṅs-lugs* and *Zur-lugs*.

After the Fifth Dalai Lama, the regent Sde-srid Saṅs-
rgyas Rgya-mtsho (1653 - 1705 A.D.) who was acquainted
with these two different schools wrote an elaborate and
authentic commentary called *Baidurya Sṅon-po*. His works
became very popular in Tibet. He also got beautiful paintings
drawn with notes on the basis of his commentary. These
beautiful paintings are more recently published in Beijing
and London.

*Rgyud-bźi* is written in the form of a dialogue between
Yid-las skyes and Rig-pa'i Ye-ses, both, the incarnations of
Lord Buddha. This work has 156 chapters comprising in
total 5900 verses and prose paragraphs. The four parts of this
work are as follows :

(1) *Rtsa-rgyud* (Root treatise) with six chapters containing
nine sections;

(2) *Bśad-rgyud* (Explanatory text) with 31 chapters
grouped into 11 sections;

(3)  *Man-nag-rgyud* (Text of instructions) with 92 chapters grouped into 15 sections; and

(4)  *Phyi-ma-rgyud* (Supplementary text) with 27 chapters grouped into four sections.

The last two chapters of the last text are of concluding nature encompassing the whole text.

The unique feature of this work is that the whole concept of medicine is described in the form of a tree having three Roots, nine Trunks, forty-seven Branches, 224 Leaves, two Flowers and three Fruits as follows:

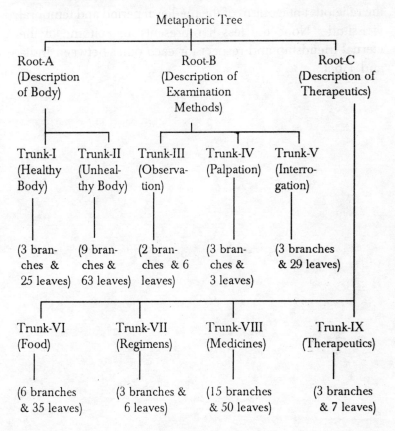

Metaphoric Tree

Root-A (Description of Body)

Root-B (Description of Examination Methods)

Root-C (Description of Therapeutics)

Trunk-I (Healthy Body) — (3 branches & 25 leaves)

Trunk-II (Unhealthy Body) — (9 branches & 63 leaves)

Trunk-III (Observation) — (2 branches & 6 leaves)

Trunk-IV (Palpation) — (3 branches & 3 leaves)

Trunk-V (Interrogation) — (3 branches & 29 leaves)

Trunk-VI (Food) — (6 branches & 35 leaves)

Trunk-VII (Regimens) — (3 branches & 6 leaves)

Trunk-VIII (Medicines) — (15 branches & 50 leaves)

Trunk-IX (Therapeutics) — (3 branches & 7 leaves)

The branches and leaves in different Trunks represent various medical topics. In addition, this metaphoric tree has two flowers representing (1) Freedom from disease, and (2) Longevity, and three fruits representing (1) Religious virtues, (2) Wealth, and (3) Happiness.

This work has undergone revisions several times, and in tune with the tradition of the medical system of the country of origin, i.e. India, it has accommodated many new drugs and recipes of the country of adaptation, i.e. Tibet. The Sanskrit original of this work is no more extant. Perhaps, like many other Sanskrit classical works, it has succumbed to the religious antagonism of the medieval period and temporal vicissitude. None the less it represents an epitome of the eternal friendship and respect for each other between India and Tibet.

# 3

# Composition of the Body

In Tibetan medicine, the individual is considered to be a microcosm, and it represents every phenomena of the macrocosm, i.e. the universe. Thus every change in the macrocosm affects the human being, and a person can bring out changes in the universe with the help of mantras or religious incantations.

The universe is composed of five basic elements (*'Byuṅ-ba*), viz., *sa, chu, me, rluṅ* and *nam-mkha'*. These philosophical terms are sometimes mistranslated as earth; water, fire, air and ether respectively keeping in view the connotations of these words in common usage. These basic elements are never found in their pure forms in the phenomenal world. In fact every substance is a conglomeration of all these five basic elements, one or other of these elements predominating the composition of the substance. This predominance of the basic elements (*'Byuṅ-ba*) produces some characteristic features in the substance as follows :

(1) The substance dominated by *Sa* basic element is characterised by heaviness, stability, dullness, smoothness, unctuousness, dryness, hardness and nourishing effect on the body;

(2) The substance dominated by *Chu* basic element is characterised by liquidity, coldness, heaviness, dullness, unctuousness, softness, moistness and smoothness;

(3) The substance dominated by *Me* basic element is characterised by heat, sharpness, dryness, roughness, lightness, unctuousness and mobility;

(4) The substance dominated by *Rluṅ* basic element is characterised by lightness, mobility, coldness, roughness, paleness, dryness, ununctuousness, quick movement and nonsliminess; and

(5) The substance dominated by *Nam-mkha'* basic element is characterised by porosity and lightness.

The body is composed of all these five basic elements which remain in a state of dynamic proportion. In their state of equilibrium, they maintain the health of an individual. If, however, because of external or internal factors, this equilibrium is disturbed, then the person suffers from diseases and even death. This disturbance in equilibrium can be corrected by supplying material through food, drinks, regimens and medicines which will increase the reduced basic elements, and reduce the increased ones. Since these basic elements are present both in the individual and in the ingredients of food, etc., and their characteristic features are known, theoretically, it appears easy to treat the diseases. But in practice, it is not so. To ascertain the exact basic element increased or decreased in the individual to cause the disease, and to determine the exact basic elements composing the ingredients of food, etc., is practically difficult.

To facilitate proper judgement, the actions of these basic elements in an individual are described in the form of three *ñes-pas* or *nads,* and the physical composition is described in the form of seven categories of *lus zuṅs* or tissue elements, and *dri-mas* or waste products which are eliminated after subserving their utility in the body. Similarly, the exact basic elements composing the ingredients of food, etc., are described in the form of *ro* or taste, *yon-tan* or attributes, *nus-pa* or potency, *zu-rjes* or the taste that emerges after digestion.

Details of these topics will be described in the succeeding chapters.

**4**

# Embryology and Anatomy

The process of conception, development of the foetus and management of the pregnant mother are described in great detail in Tibetan medicine. Tibetans believe in the existence of past-life, life after death, *las* or impressions of the past life influencing the events of the present life, and *rnam-śes* or conscious element. Accompanied with the five basic elements (*'Byuṅ-lṅa*), the conscious element impelled by the actions of its own past life which were painful, enters into the union of the unpolluted sperm (*khu*) and ovum (*khrag*) of the father and mother respectively in the uterus of the mother to cause manifestation of the embryo. This happens on the analogy of the emergence of fire by the rubbing of two pieces of wood. The characteristic features of unpolluted sperm and ovum, the morbidities developed by pollution, and their treatment are described in great detail. Characteristic features of the foetus during different weeks of pregnancy are described as follows :

(1) During the first week of the first month of pregnancy, the zygote, produced by the union of the sperm and ovum, becomes like a mixture of milk and yoghurt.

(2) During the second week, the embryo appears like a jelly having thicker consistency.

(3) During the third week, the zygote appears like curd. During this week, religious rites should be performed and medicines should be used by the mother to get the offspring of the desired sex and character. Thus,

according to Tibetan medicine, the sex of the offspring can be changed after conception and during the pregnancy;

(4) During the fourth week of pregnancy, the foetus takes different types of shape, viz., round, bi-sectional or oblong as a result of which male, female and neuter offsprings respectively are born.

(5) During the fifth week of the second month of pregnancy first of all the umblicus is formed.

(6) During the sixth week of pregnancy, the vital channel carrying the *elan vitae* is formed.

(7) During the seventh week, eyes get protruded.

(8) During the eighth week, from the trunk, the head gets protruded.

(9) During the ninth week, the body of the foetus takes appropriate shape with reference to its interior, upper and lower parts.

(10) During the tenth week, both the shoulders and hips take appropriate shape.

(11) During the eleventh week, nine orifices, viz., two eyes, two ears, two nostrils, urinary including genital tract and anus take appropriate shape.

(12) During the twelfth week, five solid visceras take appropriate shape.

(13) During the thirteenth week, six hollow visceras take appropriate shape.

(14) During the fourteenth week, the four limbs, viz., two upper limbs and two lower limbs take appropriate shape and get protruded.

(15) During the fifteenth week, two legs in the lower limb and two hands in the upper limb take appropriate shape and get protruded.

(16) During the sixteenth week, twenty fingers and toes take appropriate shape and get protruded.

(17) During the seventeenth week, the vessels connecting the external and internal organs are manifested.

(18) During the eighteenth week, muscles and fat are produced.

(19) During the nineteenth week, ligaments and tendons are produced.

(20) During the twentieth week, bones and bone-marrow are produced.

(21) During the 21st week, the skin covering the exterior of the body is produced.

(22) During the 22nd week, nine orifices representing the doors of sensory and motor organs become clear.

(23) During the 23rd week, small and big hair and nails are produced.

(24) During the 24th week, solid and hollow visceras get well developed and matured. During this period, the foetus becomes capable of feeling pain and pleasure.

(25) During the 25th week, movement of *rluṅ* takes place in the body of the foetus.

(26) During the 26th week, the memory in the mind of the foetus becomes clear.

(27) Thereafter, from the 27th to 30th week, all the parts of the foetus take clear shape.

(28) From the 31st to 35th weeks, different parts of the foetal body get more expanded. During this period, *gzi-mdaṅs* or vital essence travel between the mother and the foetus in each moment.

(29) During the 36th week and onwards, the foetus does not feel happy to remain inside the womb of the mother.

(30) During the 37th week, the foetus gets perverted thoughts.

(31) During the 38th week, the foetus turns down its head and comes out of the genital organ of the mother.

The time and process of delivery are described in great detail in the works of Tibetan medicine.

**Anatomical Descriptions**

In view of the typical way in which burials are conducted, Tibetan physicians had a good opportunity to study the anatomy of the body. The human body is composed of 360 bones which are classified into 23 groups. There are twelve large and 210 small joints, sixteen tendons, nine hundred ligaments, 21,000 hairs and eleven million hair pores. Apart from nerves, arteries, veins, lymphatic channels, 302 vital spots located in the muscles (45), fat (8), bones (32), ligaments (14), solid and hollow visceras (13) and channels of circulation (190) are described in detail. These vital spots are located in the head (62), neck (33), upper and lower parts of the trunk (95) and upper and lower limbs (112).

Apart from the tissue elements which will be described later two categories of viscera, viz., *snod* (hollow visceras) and *don* (solid visceras) are also described in detail. These visceras are as follows :

*(A) Snod or Hollow Visceras*
  (1)   *Pho-ba* or stomach;
  (2)   *Rgyu-ma* or small intestine;
  (3)   *Loṅ-ga* or large intestine;
  (4)   *Lgaṅ-pa* or urinary bladder;
  (5)   *Mkhris-thum* or gall bladder; and
  (6)   *Bsam-seu'* or reproductive organs in males and females.

*(B) Don or Solid Visceras*
  (1)   *Sñiṅ* or heart;
  (2)   *Glo-ba* or lungs;
  (3)   *Mchin-pa* or liver;
  (4)   *Mcher-pa* or spleen; and
  (5)   *Mkhal-ma* or kidneys.

Surface anatomy of these vital spots, hollow visceras and solid visceras is described in detail with diagrams of human body. The measurement of all the solid and liquid constituents of the body are also provided.

# 5

# Physiological Concepts

As has been mentioned in the fourth chapter, the body is composed of five basic elements, viz., *sa, chu, me, rluṅ* and *nam-'kha*. They remain in a state of dynamic equilibrium as the substratum of the body. They control all the functions of the body. Any disturbance in this equilibrium causes disease and death of the individual. To maintain equilibrium, the diminished ones are to be increased and the increased ones are to be reduced with the help of drugs, diet and regimens. Theoritically, it appears to be simple. But in practice, it is difficult to make out the exact condition of these elements. To facilitate proper judgement, the functional aspect of these basic elements is designated as *ñes-pa* or *nad*. The structural aspect of these basic elements is described as *lus-zuṅs*. After digestion and metabolism, the waste products which are partly used by the body and generally eliminated through the external orifices are called *dri-ma*. Since all of these are composed of the five basic elements, from these *ñes-pa, lus-zuṅs* and *dri-ma*, a physician can very easily make out their exact position and decide upon the correct treatment.

## Ñes-pa or Functional Units

All the functions of the body and mind are regulated by *ñes-pa* which is broadly classified into three categories, viz., *rluṅ, mkhris-pa* and *bad-kan*. *Rluṅ* controls and coordinates all the movements in the body. Digestion, metabolism and all other enzymatic activities in the body are controlled by *mkhris-pa*. All the liquid components and their lubricating activities in the body are controlled by *bad-kan*.

Out of these five basic elements, *nam-mkha'* and *rluṅ* enter into the composition of *rluṅ* (*rluṅ* which is the basic element is different from the *rluṅ* which is a *ñes-pa*, this is to be kept in the mind). *Me* enters into the composition of *mkhris-pa*, and *chu* as well as *sa* enter into the composition of *bad-kan*.

Because of their composing basic elements, these three *ñes-pas* exhibit characteristic attributes as follows :

*Attributes of Rluṅ*

(1)  Ununctuousness (*rtsub*);
(2)  Lightness (*yaṅ-ba*);
(3)  Coldness (*graṅ-ba*);
(4)  Subtleness (*phra*);
(5)  Coarseness (*sra*); and
(6)  Mobility (*g'yo-ba*).

*Attributes of Mkhris-pa*

(1)  Sharpness (*rno*);
(2)  Hot (*tsha*);
(3)  Lightness (*yaṅ*);
(4)  Foul smell like washing of flesh (*dri-mñam*);
(5)  Fluidity ('*khru*);
(6)  Liquidity (*gśer-ba*); and
(7)  Slightly unctuous (*snum-bcas*).

*Attributes of Bad-kan*

(1)  Unctuousness (*snum*);
(2)  Coldness in excess (*bsil-ba*);
(3)  Heaviness (*lci*);

(4)   Dullness (*rtul*);
(5)   Smoothness (*'jam*);
(6)   Stability (*brtan*); and
(7)   Sliminess ('*byar-bag-can*).

These three *ñes-pas* perform the following activities in general :

## Functions of Rluṅ in General

*Rluṅ*, in general, performs the following activities in the body :

(1)   Controls inspiration and expiration;
(2)   Produces enthusiasm;
(3)   Controls all the movements in the body;
(4)   Helps in the manifestation of different urges (for micturition, defecation, etc.,) in the body;
(5)   Maintains sharpness (clarity) of the sense organs; and
(6)   Helps in the proper transmission (movement) of the nutrients to the tissue elements.

## Functions of Mkhris-pa in General

*Mkhris-pa,* in general, performs the following activities in the body :

(1)   Produces hunger and thirst;
(2)   Promotes the desire to take food and helps in its digestion as well as metabolism;
(3)   Produces heat and clear complexion in the body; and
(4)   Helps in the exhibition of bravery and production of intellect.

## Functions of Bad-kan in General

*Bad-kan*, in general, performs the following activities in the body :

(1) Produces stability of the body and the mind;

(2) Induces sleep;

(3) Promotes compactness of the joints;

(4) Increases the capacity to forgive others for their mistakes; and

(5) Causes softness and unctuousness of the body.

## Divisions of Ñes-pas

Each of these three *ñes-pas* is again subdivided into five categories depending upon their location and specific functions.

*(A) Five Divisions of Rluṅ*

Five divisions of *rluṅ* are as follows :

(1) *Srog-'dzin* :

It is located in the upper part of the body, viz., neck and chest, and it performs the following functions :

(a) Helps in the deglutition of food and drinks;

(b) Helps in breathing, spitting, sneezing and eructations;

(c) Promotes the sharpness of wisdom and sense perception; and

(d) Controls the mind.

(2) *Gyen-du-rgyu*

It is located in the chest, and it moves among the nose, tongue and throat. It performs the following functions :

(a) Helps in the production of speech;

(b) Helps in making efforts; and

(c) Promotes energy, complexion, strength and clarity of memory.

(3) *Khyab-byed*

It is located in the heart and moves all over the body. It's functions are as follows :

It helps a person to lift a substance upwards or press it downwards. It also helps in motions, extension, contraction and other activities like opening and closing of the eyes.

(4)  *Me-dań-mñam-pa*

It is located in the stomach, and moves throughout the gastro-intestinal tract. Its functions are as follows :

(a) Digestion of food;

(b) Separation of chyle from the stool; and

(c) Formation of stool.

(5)  *Thur-du-sel*

It is located in the pelvic region, and moves inside the colon, urinary bladder, genital organs and thighs. It controls (helps) the ejaculation of semen, menstrual secretion (including ovum), stool, urine and foetus during delivery.

*(B) Five Divisions of Mkhris-pa*

*Mkhris-pa* is of five types, and their locations as well as functions are as follows :

(1)  *'Ju byed*

This is located inside the intestines and stomach. Its functions are as follows :

(a) Helps in the digestion of food;

(b) Separates chyle from the digested food stuff;

(c) Produces heat in the body; and

(d) Nourishes and provides strength to the remaining four types of *mkhris-pa*.

(2)  *Mdańs-sgyur*

It is located in the liver. It imparts colour to chyle, thus helping in blood formation.

(3)  *Sgrub byed*

It is located in the heart. It is responsible for the manifestation of intellect, ego and wisdom. It helps in the satisfaction of the mental desires.

(4) *Mthon-byed*

It is located in the eyes. It is responsible for the perception of vision.

(5) *Mdog-gsal*

It is located in the skin, and it imparts colour to it (skin).

## (C) Five Divisions of Bad-kan

*Bad-kan* is of five types, and their locations as well as functions are as follows :

(1) *Rten-byed*

It is located in the chest. It gives support to the other varieties of *bad-kan*. It performs the functions of water.

(2) *Myag-byed*

It is located in the stomach. It helps in the preparation of dough of the ingested food and drinks. It also helps in the breaking of these ingredients into small particles.

(3) *Myon-byed*

It is located in the tongue. It helps in the gustatory perception.

(4) *Tshim-byed*

It is located in the head. It provides nourishment to sense organs.

(5) *'Byor-byed*

It is located in all the joints. It helps in greasing, contraction and expansion of these joints.

## Lus-zuns or Tissue Elements

These five basic elements also enter into the structure of the body in the form of tissue elements. These are of seven categories as follows :

(1) *Daṅs-ma* or the plasma including chyle;
(2) *Khrag* or blood (specially the haemoglobin fraction in the red blood cells);
(3) *Śa* or muscle tissue;
(4) *Tshil* or fat tissue;
(5) *Rus-pa* or bone tissue including cartilages;
(6) *Rkaṅ* or bone marrow; and
(7) *Khu* or semen in males and ovum in the females.

These tissue elements are responsible for the sustenance of the body. These are composed of all the five categories of basic elements. However, *chu* is an important constituent of plasma and semen; *sa* is predominant in the muscle tissues and bones; *me* is predominant in the bone-marrow and blood; and the porosity in the bone is caused by the *rluṅ* and *nam-'kha.* From the increase or decrease of these tissue elements, a physician can determine the status of the five basic elements in the body.

## Dri-ma or Waste-Products

During the process of digestion and metabolism, several by-products come out. They do have some useful function in the body. But ultimately most of these waste products get eliminated from the body. There are three important waste products, viz., stool (*bsaṅ*), urine (*gcin*) and sweat (*rṅul*). Increase or decrease of these and such other waste products lead to several diseases. These waste products are also composed of five basic elements.

## Solid and Hollow Visceras

For the maintenance of body physiology, there are several visceral organs, which are constituted of these tissue elements. These are broadly classified into two categories, viz., *don* or solid visceras and *snod* or hollow visceras. Solid visceras are five in number, viz., heart, liver, lungs, spleen and kidneys. Hollow visceras are six in number, viz., stomach, small intestine, large intestine, gall bladder, urinary bladder and reproductive organs. Functions of these visceras are described in detail in the texts on Tibetan medicine.

## Digestion and Metabolism

The tissues of the body undergo diminution every moment as a part of the process of living. In the young age, the tissues increase in quantity. The lost tissue elements are replenished, and these are made to grow in infancy and adulthood through food and drinks. But the ingredients of food and drinks are not homologous to the tissues. There is, therefore, a need for their digestion and metabolism. The enzymes responsible for this action are called *me-drod*. It is of four types as follows :

(1) *Mi-sñoms* or irregular; this is called by the aggravation of *rluṅ*;

(2) *Rno-ba* or sharp; this is caused by the aggravation of *mkhris-pa*;

(3) *Chuṅ* or dull; this is caused by the aggravation of *bad-kan*; and

(4) *Mñam-pa* or harmoneous; this is caused by the equilibrium of all the three *ñes-pas*.

The fourth type of *me-drod* is very useful for good health, and a person should always try to maintain it with appropriate food, drinks and regimens. The first three types of *me-drod* give rise to several diseases.

This *me-drod* (or group of enzymes) is again divided into thirteen categories depending upon the place of their location and specific functions. One group is located in the gastro-intestinal tract, and it helps in the digestion of food.

Five groups are located in the liver, and they help in converting nonhomologous nutrients (composed of five basic elements) into homologous ones. Besides, there are seven groups of *me-drod* (enzymes) which are located in the tissue-elements, and they help in the synthesis of seven categories of tissues from the nutrient fluid which is absorbed into the blood-stream after the digestion of the food.

## Process of Digestion

In the beginning, the ingested food and drinks which are of six different tastes become sticky by the action of *myag-byed* type of *bad-kan*. The end product of this reaction becomes sweet in taste. Thereafter, by the action of *'ju-byed* type of *mkhris-pa*, the food stuff becomes further digested, and the end product becomes sour in taste. At the end, by the action of *me-mñam* type of *rluṅ*, the nourishing part of the food gets absorbed into the blood stream from the intestine. The remaining stuff in the colon becomes pungent in taste which comes out from the rectum in the form of stool.

## Process of Metabolism

From the intestine, the nutrient part of the food gets absorbed in the form of chyle and goes to the liver. In the liver, the chyle gets converted into blood. This blood becomes transformed into muscle tissue by the reaction of *me-drod* (enzymes). The muscle tissue, thereafter, gets converted into fat, fat into bone, bone into bone-marrow, and bone-marrow into semen (in males) and ovum (in females) by the enzymes (*me-drod*) specific to each of these tissue elements. This metabolic process gives rise to several byproducts (waste products).

## By-products of Digestion and Metabolism

The by-products of digestion and metabolism are as follows :

(1) Stool and urine are the waste products of food during the process of digestion;

(2) Phlegm is the by-product of chyle;

(3) Bile is the by-product of blood;

(4) Excreta from the orifices of the body are the by-products of muscle tissue;

(5) The greasy material in the body is the by-product of fat;

(6) Teeth, nails and hair are the by-products of bone; and

(7) The unctuous material in the stool is the by-product of bone-marrow.

Some of these by-products remain in the body for some time, and serve some useful purpose. But most of these are excreted out of the body as waste product.

## Mdaṅs-ma or Vital Essence

The essence of all these tissue elements is called *mdaṅs-ma* (vital essence), and it is responsible for making the body endowed with excellent complexion. Its diminution or change in its composition leads to several obstinate diseases and even death.

## Lto-ba or Bowel Movement

Proper bowel movement is considered essential for good health of an individual. It is of three types as follows :

(1) *Sra-la* or costive bowel; this is caused by the aggravation of *rluṅ*;

(2)  *Sñi* or loose bowel; this is caused by the aggravation of *mkhris-pa*; and

(3)  *Bar-mar* or moderate; this is caused by the aggravation of *bad-kan*, and also by the state of equilibrium of all the *ñes-pas*.

While examining a patient, the Tibetan physician always enquiries about the condition of the bowel movement and prescribes medicines accordingly.

## Classification of the Body

The body of the individual is classified according to sex, age, psycho-somatic constitution and state of the *ñes-pas*. On the basis of sex, persons are classified into three categories, viz., male (*pho*), female (*mo*); and neuter (*ma-niṅ*). On the basis of age, persons are classified into three categories, viz., *byis-pa* or infant (up to the age of sixteen years), *dar-ma* or adult (up to the age of seventy years), and *rgan-po* or old (after the age of seventy years till the death). On the basis of the state of the *ñes-pas*, the individuals are classified into two categories, viz., *rnam-par ma gyur* or a healthy person without any disease and *rnam-gyur* or a diseased person.

## Raṅ-bźin or Psycho-Somatic Constitution

At the time of conception (union of the sperm and ovum), the *ñes-pa* aggravated in the womb of the mother determines the *raṅ-bźin* or psycho-somatic constitution of the individual. The specific features acquired by the individual during this time continue till death. Tibetan physicians always keep these features of the patient in view while treating him. Even for an apparently healthy person, they provide some dos and don'ts in the form of food, drinks and regimens for the preservation and promotion of their positive health on the basis of this *raṅ-bźin* or psycho-somatic constitution.

*Raṅ-bźin* cr constitution is of seven types depending upon the aggravation of *rluṅ, mkhris-pa, bad-kan, rluṅ* and *mkhris-pa, rluṅ* and *bad-kan, mkhris-pa* and *bad-kan* and equilibrium of all the three *ñes-pas* at the time of conception.

## Rluṅ Type of Constitution

A person having *rluṅ* type of *raṅ-bźin* or constitution has the following characteristic features :

(1)  His physique is crooked;
(2)  He is emaciated and thin;
(3)  He is grayish in colour;
(4)  He is talkative;
(5)  He is incapable of tolerating exposure to the cold;
(6)  While walking different types of sound are produced in his joints;
(7)  He has less of wealth;
(8)  His span of life is too short;
(9)  He sleeps less;
(10) Structurally, his body is small;
(11) He is fond of songs, jokes, quarrel, women and hunting;
(12) He likes food and drinks which are sweet, sour, saline and pungent in taste; and
(13) He bears the characteristic features of vultures, crows and foxes.

## Mkhris-pa Type of Constitution

A person having *mkhris-pa* type of *raṅ-bźin* or constitution has the following characteristic features :

(1)  He is always hungry and thirsty;

(2)    His hair and body are yellow in colour;

(3)    He has sharp intellect and more of ego;

(4)    He has excess of sweating and putrid odour emanates from his body;

(5)    He has moderate span of life, wealth and body-size;

(6)    He likes food ingredients which are sweet, bitter, astringent and cold; and

(7)    He bears characteristic features of tiger, monkey and *gnod-spyin* (a group of celestial spirits).

## Bad-kan Type of Constitution

A person having *bad-kan* type of *raṅ-bźin* or constitution has the following characteristic features :

(1)    His body is cold to touch;

(2)    His bones and joints are compact;

(3)    He has more of flesh in the body;

(4)    He is white in colour;

(5)    He has power to tolerate hunger, thirst, pain and exposure to heat;

(6)    He is fatty;

(7)    He lives a long span of life;

(8)    He possesses more of wealth, and he sleeps for a long time and very deeply;

(9)    His anger and enmity last long;

(10)   By nature, he likes to make donations, and he is very gentle by nature;

(11)   He desires to take food, ingredients of which are pungent, sour, astringent and unctuous; and

(12)   He possesses the characteristic features of lion and bull.

Permutation and combination of these features characterise the *raṅ-bźin* or constitution of the remaining types of persons. Of these, the person having *rluṅ* type of *raṅ-bźin* (constitution caused by the aggravation of *rluṅ* at the time of conception) is inferior; the person having *mkhris-pa* type of *raṅ-bźin* (constitution caused by the aggravation of *mkhris-pa* at the time of conception) is medium, and the person having *bad-kan* type of *raṅ-bźin* (constitution caused by the aggravation of *bad-kan* at the time of conception) is superior. If all these three types of *ñes-pa* are in a state of equilibrium at the time of conception, then the *raṅ-bźin* (constitution) caused thereby is of excellent nature. The constitutions caused by the aggravation of two of these three *ñes-pas* during conception are of moderate nature.

During examination of a patient, from the signs, symptoms, pulse and urine examination, the physician ascertains the nature of the *ñes-pas* which are then aggravated. Simultaneously, the *ñes-pa* which is responsible for the manifestation of a particular type of *raṅ-bźin* in the patient at the time of conception is determined. But this needs detailed examination, and acquaintance with the patient right from his childhood.

# 6

# Pathological Concepts

According to Tibetan medicine, diseases are caused by two categories of etiological factors, viz., effects of the actions of the past life (*sṅon gyi las*) and effects of *ñes-pas* aggravated as a result of food, regimens, etc., in the present life (*tshe 'di'i ñes*). Buddhism firmly believes in the existence of the past-life and life after death. This process of rebirth continues till a person reaches Buddhahood by his virtuous acts, religious practices and spiritual elevation after which he gets salvation. One can reach this state of salvation and still continue his mundane activities for the benefit of other sentient creatures. Impressions of his noble activities then do not afflict him, and he becomes free from the whirl of life and death.

The etiological factors of the present life are of two categories, viz., *rgyu* or primary cause and *rkyen* or secondary causes. The *rgyu* or primary cause is again of two types as follows :

(1) *Riṅ-rgyu* or distant cause; and
(2) *Ñe-rgyu* or immediate cause.

The distant cause of all diseases in general is *ma-rig* or ignorance which is specifically manifested in the form of *'dod chags* or passion, *źe-ldaṅ* or anger and *gti-mug* or illusion. All living beings suffer from these distant causes. However, those who could overcome these factors by their religious practices do not succumb to diseases.

The immediate cause of all diseases is the aggravation of three *ñes-pas*, viz., *rluṅ*, *mkhris-pa* and *bad-kan*, the nature of which has already been discussed. These three *ñes-pas* are closely related to the three distant causes, inasmuch as *rluṅ* is caused by *'dod-chags* or passion, *mkhris-pa* is caused by *że-ldaṅ* or anger, and *bad-kan* is caused by *gti-mug* or illusion.

*Rluṅ, mkhris-pa* and *bad-kan* normally remain in a state of equilibrium in a healthy person. But because of unwholesome diet, drinks, regimens and seasonal effects, they get either diminished (in quantity or quality) or aggravated. These aggravated *ñes-pas* cause diseases by vitiating the tissue elements (*lus-zuṅs*) or waste products (*dri-ma*). Apart from these endogenous causes, a disease may also be caused by exogenous causes like injury, affliction by poisons and evil spirits. (Tibetan medicine believes in the existence of the evil spirits, and there is a special branch of this medical system to treat such diseases). These exogenous factors ultimately produce a disease in which process the *ñes-pas* get naturally aggravated.

For producing a malady, these *nes-pas* undergo four morbid stages, viz., accumulation (*gsog*), aggravation (*ldaṅ*), spreading (*'phel-ba*) and localisation (*brten-pa'i gnas*). In this location which may be either solid viscera or hollow viscera or tissue element or waste product, the disease is manifested to produce different signs and symptoms.

Each disease, depending the process of pathogenesis, produces different signs and symptoms, and these are described in the medical texts. The physician examines them to diagnose the disease and to suggest therapeutic measures for its cure. The signs and symptoms produced by the aggravation of these three *ñes-pas* are as follows :

*Signs and Symptoms of Aggravated Rluṅ*

(1)  Emaciation, black coloration and desire for warm things;

(2)  Trembling of the body, flatulence and constipation;
(3)  Delirium and giddiness; and
(4)  Diminution of strength, sleep and sense perception.

### Signs and Symptoms of Aggravated Mkhris-pa

(1)  Yellow coloration of the stool, urine, skin and eyes;
(2)  Excessive hunger and thirst;
(3)  Burning sensation in the body; and
(4)  Loss of sleep and diarrhoea.

### Signs and Symptoms of Aggravated Bad-kan

(1)  Suppression of the power of digestion and metabolism, and indigestion of food;
(2)  Heaviness of the body, white coloration of the skin, and laziness as well as slothness of the limbs; and
(3)  Excessive salivation, coughing, sleep and dyspnoea.

Though the knowledge of the signs and symptoms of aggravated *ñes-pas* is important for successful diagnosis and treatment of diseases, it is also necessary for the physician to be acquainted with the signs and symptoms of the diminished ones which are as follows :

### Signs and Symptoms of Diminished Rluṅ

If *rluṅ* is diminished then there is lassitude, loss of power to talk, uneasy feeling in the body, loss of memory and appearance of the signs and symptoms of aggravated *bad-kan*.

### Signs and Symptoms of Diminished Mkhris-pa

If *mkhris-pa* is diminished, then there is diminution in the power of digestion and the metabolic process becomes slow. The body complexion is changed as a result of which it becomes black and cold.

## Signs and Symptoms of Diminished Bad-kan

If *bad-kan* is diminished, then the person feels emptiness in the locations of *bad-kan*. In addition, there is giddiness, palpitation and losseness of the joints.

The signs and symptoms described above pertain to the increase or decrease in the quantity of *rluṅ, mkhris-pa* and *bad-kan*. Besides, these *ñes-pas* undergo qualitative changes, i.e. their attributes undergo morbid changes which is called *'khrugs* or vitiation. The signs and symptoms produced as a result of this vitiation of *ñes-pas* are as follows :

## Signs and Symptoms of Vitiated Rluṅ

(1) The pulse appears as if the physician's fingers are placed over an empty leather bag or there is a feeling as if the pulse is swimming or swinging;

(2) The urine looks like water and lustreless. When struck with a stick, it appears to be thin and slow in moving. When the urine poured from one pot to another during examination, more of bubbles and less of froth appear;

(3) There is slight giddiness in the head and noise appears in the ears;

(4) The tongue is dry, red coloured and unctuous, and there is astringent taste in the mouth;

(5) There is colic pain which moves from one place to the other, cold shivering, pain in the back and lassitude;

(6) There is rigidity, shrivelling, breaking sensation and a feeling as if the body is pulled out and twisted;

(7)   There is trembling, excess of pain, horripilation and breaking as well as expansion of bones and cartilages;

(8)   There is sleeplessness, yawning, shivering, desire to stretch the body and burning sensation while taking food;

(9)   There is a feeling as if the pelvic region, lumber region and all bones as well as joints are contracted;

(10)  There is pricking pain at the back of the neck, chest, temples and sides of the chest;

(11)  While passing stool and flatus, the anus remains wide open, and there is pressure as well as pain in the anal region;

(12)  There is vomiting without any substance coming out, and in the morning the patient spits out frothy saliva;

(13)  There is gurgling sound in the upper part of the abdomen; and

(14)  The ailments get aggravated during early part of the morning (dawn), later part of the day (evening) and after the digestion of food.

## Signs and Symptoms of Vitiated Mkhris Bad-kan-pa

(1)   The pulse is thin in volume, fast and swift;

(2)   The urine becomes red or yellow in colour, and there is excess of smell, warmth and vapour;

(3)   There is headache, sloughing of the muscle tissue, and bitter as well as sour taste in the mouth;

(4)   There is a thick coating of phlegm over the tongue, and dryness of the nostrils;

(5)   The eyes become cloudy, red or yellow. There is pain in the eyes, and eye-lids adhere together because of sticky exudation;

(6)   There is less of sleep at night and no sleep during the day time;

(7) The phlegm becomes red or yellow in colour and pungent in taste;

(8) There is bleeding from different parts of the body. There is excess of thirst and sweating which is foul smelling;

(9) The colour of the skin is either red or yellow; and

(10) The ailment gets aggravated during mid-day, mid-night and during the process of digestion of food.

## Signs and Symptoms of Vitiated Mkhris-pa

(1) The pulse is hidden, difficult to locate and dull;

(2) The urine is white in colour, and there is less of smell and vapour in it;

(3) Offensive smell comes out of the mouth. The tongue and gums are pale, the eyes are white and swollen;

(4) More of nasal secretion and phlegm;

(5) Confusion in the mind and heaviness in the head and body;

(6) Loss of appetite and less power of digestion and metabolism;

(7) Pain in the kidney region, lumber region, oedema in the body and appearance of goiter;

(8) Throwing out of food and phlegm while vomiting, and diarrhoea;

(9) Dullness of memory, excess of sleep and laziness;

(10) Itching, stiffness and compactness of joints, and swelling of muscles;

(11) Delay in the manifestation and progress of diseases; and

(12) Aggravation of the ailment during heavy rain, morning, evening and before the onset of the digestion of food.

Like *ñes-pas*, the tissue elements (*lus-zuñs*) and waste products (*dri-ma*) undergo morbid changes in the form of increase ('*phel*) or decrease (*zad*) in their quantity producing characteristic signs and symptoms which are as follows :

*Signs and Symptoms of Increased Plasma*

Increase of *dañs-ma* (plasma and chyle) produces signs and symptoms like those of aggravated *bad-kan*, viz., suppression of the power of digestion and metabolism, heaviness of the body, white coloration of the body, laziness, slothness of the limbs, excessive salivation, coughing, excessive sleep and dyspnoea.

*Signs and Symptoms of Diminished Plasma*

If *dañsa-ma* (plasma including chyle) is diminished, then there is dryness of the muscles, difficulty in swallowing of food, dryness of the skin and inability to tolerate loud noise.

*Signs and Symptoms of Increased Blood*

If *khrag* (blood, specifically the red-fraction of it) is increased, then there is manifestation of diseases like erysipelas, internal abscess, splenic disorder, obstinate skin diseases including leprosy, phantom tumour, bleeding from different parts of the body and jaundice.

*Signs and Symptoms of Diminished Blood*

If blood is diminished, then there is emptiness in the vessels, dryness of the skin and liking for cold things.

### Signs and Symptoms of Increased Muscle Tissue

If *śa* or muscle tissue is increased, then the person suffers from goiter, tumours and muscular growth.

### Signs and Symptoms of Diminished Muscle Tissue

If *śa* or muscle tissue is diminished, then the person suffers from pain in the joints and limbs, and adherance of the skin to the bones.

### Signs and Symptoms of Increased Fat

If *tshil* or fat is increased, then the person suffers from fatigue and appearance of excess fat in the breasts and abdomen.

### Signs and Symptoms of Diminished Fat

If *tshil* or fat is diminished, then the person suffers from insomnia, dryness of the muscles and pale-green coloration of the skin.

### Signs and Symptoms of Increased Bone-Tissue

If *rus-pa* or bone-tissue is increased, then the person suffers from tumours in the bone and formation of extra teeth.

### Signs and Symptoms of Diminished Bone-Tissue

If *rus-pa* or bone-tissue is diminished, then the person suffers from hair-fall, and falling of teeth and nail.

### Signs and Symptoms of Increased Bone-Marrow

If *rkaṅ* or bone-marrow is increased, then the person

suffers from heaviness of the body and eyes, appearance of carbuncles and swellings in the finger-joints and toes.

### Signs and Symptoms of Diminished Bone-Marrow

If *rkaṅ* or bone-marrow is diminished, then the person suffers from the feeling of emptiness inside the bones, giddiness and appearance of darkness before the eyes.

### Signs and Symptoms of Increased Semen

If *khu-ba* or semen is increased, then the person suffers from calculus in the seminal channel and excessive sexual desire.

### Signs and Symptoms of Diminished Semen

If *khu-ba* or semen is diminished, then the person suffers from bleeding and burning sensation along with ejaculation of semen.

### Signs and Symptoms of Increased Stool

If *bśaṅ* or stool is increased in quantity, then the person suffers from heaviness of the body, flatulence and gurgling sound in the intestine.

### Signs and Symptoms of Diminished Stool

If *bśaṅ* or stool is diminished, then the person suffers from gurgling sound in the intestine and their twisting. There will be upward movement of the flatus inside the intestine and pain in the sides of the chest as well as cardiac region.

*Signs and Symptoms of Increased Urine*

If *gcin* or urine is increased in quantity, then the person suffers from pain in the urinary bladder and a feeling as if he has not passed urine even after urination.

*Signs and Symptoms of Diminished Urine*

If *gcin* or urine is diminished, then the person suffers from decoloration of urine, hematuria and anuria.

*Signs and Symptoms of Increased Sweat*

If *rṅul* or sweat is increased, then the person suffers from excessive sweating, foul smell of the body and appearance of skin diseases.

*Signs and Symptoms of Diminished Sweat*

If *rṅul* or sweat is diminished, then the person suffers from cracking of the skin, horripilation and depilation of hair.

*Mdaṅs or Vital Essence*

*Mdaṅs* represents the essence of all the tissue elements in the body. It is responsible for complexion and immunity of the body against the attacks of diseases. If this substance is diminished in quantity or quality, then the person suffers from fear, emaciation, timidity, weakness, sorrow and dullness of complexion.

## Suppression of Manifested Natural Urges

For the manifestation of endogenous diseases impairement of or morbidity in the *drod* (enzymes responsible for digestion and metabolism) is the *sine-qua-non*. This causes the formation of uncooked material which circulates in the body, and gets lodged in a channel of circulation. Thereafter, the pathogenic process for the manifestation of the disease starts. This morbidity in the *drod* is caused by unwholesome food, drinks, regimens and seasonal effects. One of the important factors for causing this morbidity is the suppression of naturally manifested urges (*sugs-bgag*). These natural urges are of thirteen types and their suppression causes the following ailments :

### (1) *Suppression of the Urge of Hunger*

If the manifested urge for taking food (appetite) is suppressed (*bkres-bkag*), then the person suffers from malaise, emaciation, anorexia and giddiness.

### (2) *Suppression of the Urge of Thirst*

If the urge of thirst is suppressed (*skom-bkag*), then the person suffers from dryness of the mouth, giddiness, heart diseases and unconsciousness.

### (3) *Suppression of the Urge for Vomiting*

If the manifested urge for vomiting is suppressed (*skyugs-bkag*), then this gives rise to nausea, dyspnoea, anemia, erysipelas, itching, urticaria, obstinate skin diseases including leprosy, eye diseases, coughing and infectious fever.

## (4) *Suppression of the Urge for Sneezing*

If the manifested urge for sneezing is suppressed (*sbrid-bkag*), then this gives rise to lack of clarity in the sense perception, headache, torticolis and facial paralysis.

## (5) *Suppression of the Urge for Yawning*

If the manifested urge for yawning is suppressed (*g'yal-bkag*), then this gives rise to the same ailments as mentioned above.

## (6) *Suppression of the Urge for Deep-Breathing*

If the manifested urge for deep-breathing is suppressed (*ñal-dub-dbugs bkag*), then this gives rise to phantom tumour, heart diseases and unconsciousness.

## (7) *Suppression of the Urge for Sleep*

If the manifested urge for sleep is suppressed (*gñid-bkag*), then this gives rise to excessive yawning, laziness, heaviness of the head, tiredness of the eyes and indigestion.

## (8) *Suppression of the Urge for Coughing*

If the manifested urge for coughing is suppressed (*lud-pa-bkag*), then this gives rise to excessive coughing, dyspnoea, emaciation, hiccups, heart diseases and anorexia.

## (9) *Suppression of the Urge for Weeping*

If the manifested urge for weeping is suppressed (*mchil-*

*ma-bkag*), then this gives rise to heart diseases, head diseases, chronic cold, giddiness and anorexia.

## (10) *Suppression of the Urge for Voiding Flatus*

If the manifested urge for voiding flatus is suppressed (*'phyen-bkag*), then this gives rise to upward movement of abdominal air, obstruction to the passage of flatus and stool, phantom tumour, colic pain, reduction in the sharpness of eye-sight, suppression of the power of digestion and heart diseases.

## (11) *Suppression of the Urge for Voiding Stool*

If the manifested urge for voiding stool is suppressed (*bśan-ba-bkag*), then this gives rise to diseases of the head, excretion of the impure material or stool through the mouth, pain in the calf region and chronic cold.

## (12) *Suppression of the Urge for Urination*

If the manifested urge for urination is suppressed (*gcin-bkag*), then this gives rise to stone in the urinary tract, pain in the region of urinary bladder, pain in the penis and pain in the pelvic region.

## (13) *Suppression of the Urge for Seminal Ejaculation*

If the manifested urge for seminal ejaculation is suppressed (*khu-ba bkag*), then this gives rise to excessive ejaculation of semen, diseases of penis, anuria, calculus in the genito-urinary tract, scrotal enlargement and impotency.

Suppression of these naturally manifested urges should,

therefore, be strictly avoided if a person wants to lead a healthy and happy life. Inducing these natural urges when these are not manifested also causes diseases. This happens because of the aggravation of the *rluṅ* by such artificial and forceful inducement.

# 7

# Pharmacological Concepts

Tibetan medicine has its unique concepts of drug-composition and drug-action which elucidate the rationality of therapeutics. Without this knowledge, use of recipes simply from their indications does not lead to much success.

As has been described before, the human body is composed of five basic elements, and any disturbance in their equilibrium causes disease and decay. To restore this balance or equilibrium the increased elements are to be reduced and the diminished ones are to be increased by the appropriate administration of drugs, diet, drinks and regimens. Characteristic features of drugs, etc., dominated by these five basic elements are described as follows :

*Attributes of Drugs Dominated by Sa*

    (1)   *Lci* or heaviness;
    (2)   *Brtan* or stability;
    (3)   *Rtul* or dullness;
    (4)   *'Jam* or smoothness;
    (5)   *Snum* or unctuousness;
    (6)   *Skam* or dryness;
    (7)   *Mkhran* or hardness; and
    (8)   *Brtas* or nourishing effect.

*Attributes of Drugs Dominated by Chu*

    (1)   *Sla* or liquidity;

(2)   *Bsil* or coldness;
(3)   *Lci* or heaviness;
(4)   *Rtul* or dullness;
(5)   *Snum* or unctuousness;
(6)   *Mñen* or softness;
(7)   *Brlan* or moistness; and
(8)   *'Jam* or smoothness.

## Attributes of Drugs Dominated by Me

(1)   *Tsha* or hot;
(2)   *Rno* or sharpness;
(3)   *Skam* or dryness;
(4)   *Rtsub* or roughness;
(5)   *Yaṅ* or lightness;
(6)   *Snum* or unctuousness; and
(7)   *Gyo* or mobility.

## Attributes of Drugs Dominated by Rluṅ

(1)   *Yaṅ* or lightness;
(2)   *Gyo* or mobility;
(3)   *Graṅ* or coldness;
(4)   *Rtsub* or roughness;
(5)   *Skya* or paleness;
(6)   *Skam* or dryness;
(7)   *Sra* or ununctuousness;
(8)   *Bskyod* or movement; and
(9)   *Khyab-byed* or nonsliminess.

## Attributes of Drugs Dominated by Nam-mkha'

Drugs dominated by the basic element *nam-mkha'* have
the attributes of all the four types of ingredients described

before. They are characterised by porosity and lightness.
They provide space to other four types of ingredients.

From the above description, it will be seen that number
of attributes are shared by these five categories of basic
elements because of which it becomes difficult for an ordinary
physician to select and administer them appropriately. To
facilitate, the predominance of these basic elements is
described in the form of *ro* or taste, *zu-rjes* or the taste that
arises after the digestion of the drug, and *nus-pa* or potency.

## Ro or Taste

*Ro* or tastes are of six types, viz., *mṅar* or sweet, *skyur* or
sour, *lan-tsha* or saline, *kha* or bitter, *tsha* or pungent and
*bska* or astringent. Of these, the former ones are better
promoters of life and strength than the latter ones. One can
observe these tastes by tongue.

From these tastes the physician can easily identify the
predominance of basic elements (*'byuṅ*) in an ingredient of
drug and diet as follows :

| Taste | Dominating Basic Elements |
|---|---|
| (1) Sweet | *sa* and *chu* |
| (2) Sour | *me* and *sa* |
| (3) Saline | *chu* and *me* |
| (4) Bitter | *chu* and *rluṅ* |
| (5) Pungent | *me* and *rluṅ* |
| (6) Astringent | *sa* and *rluṅ* |

*Attributes of Sweet Taste*

Sweet taste causes stickiness in the mouth, and it is
relishing.

### Attributes of Sour Taste

Sour taste causes tingling sensation in the teeth, is exceedingly pleasing and causes salivation.

### Attributes of Saline Taste

Saline ingredients cause burning sensation and exudation of liquids from the place where they come in contact with.

### Attributes of Bitter Taste

Ingredients having bitter taste take out sticky material from the mouth. They also help in the cleansing pus, etc., from any part of the body. They inhibit excessive appetite.

### Attributes of Pungent Taste.

Ingredients having pungent taste cause irritation in the mouth and tongue to cause salivation. They also cause lachrimation.

### Attributes of Astringent Taste

Ingredients having astringent taste cause numbness of the tongue and throat. They produce dryness and choking sensation.

Since all the material in this phenomenal world are composed of all the five basic elements in different proportions, it is difficult to find a substance having absolutely one taste. A substance is called sweet, sour, etc., because of the predominance of these tastes. A substance may have one or more tastes predominantely manifested. Ingredients of drug and diet dominated by one of these tastes are grouped and illustrated as follows :

### Group of Sweet Drugs

Liquorice, grapes, saffron, bamboo-mana, *Cassia fistula*, asparagus, sugar, jaggery, honey, meat, ghee and such other drugs belong to the group having sweet taste.

### Group of Sour Drugs

Pomegranate, apple, *Emblica officinalis*, ber fruit, yoghurt, butter-milk, alcoholic drinks, vinegar and such other ingredients belong to the group having sour taste.

### Group of Saline Drugs

Different types of salt like sea-salt, rock-salt, black-salt, salt collected from the earth, salt prepared from horns and ash of plants, Sodium bicarbonate and Potassium bicarbonate belong to this group.

### Group of Bitter Drugs

*Picrorhiza kurroa, Azadirachta indica* (neem tree), *Aconitum heterophylum, Hollarrhena antidysenterica,* musk, different types of bile collected from animals, curcuma, *Adhatoda vasica, śilājīta* (exudate from stones) and such other ingredients belong to this group.

### Group of Pungent Drugs

Black pepper, ginger, long pepper, asafoetida, onion, garlic and such other drugs belong to this group.

*Group of Astringent Drugs*

Sandal wood, *Terminalia chebula, Terminalia belerica*, lotus and such other drugs belong to this category.

*Therapeutic Action of Different Tastes*

As has been described before, the five basic elements are represented in the human body in the form of three *ñes-pas*, viz., *rluñ, mkhris-pa* and *bad-kan* whose attributes and functions are already described. These five basic elements also enter into the composition of the ingredients of drugs, diet and drinks to produce different types of tastes. Thus, it becomes easy to identify the ingredients and administer them to the patient to correct his ailments caused by the disturbance of equilibrium of basic elements. The actions of different tastes on the three *ñes-pas* are as follows :

(1)  Sweet, sour, saline and pungent tastes alleviate *rluñ*;

(2)  Bitter, sweet and astringent tastes alleviate *mkhris-pa*; and

(3)  Pungent, sour and saline tastes alleviate *bad-kan*.

Apart from actions on the three *ñes-pas*, these ingredients having different tastes also affect the tissue elements and other physiological functions of the body. If consumed in excess, they may give rise to several diseases which are described below :

*Action of Ingredient Having Sweet Taste*

(1)  It is wholesome;

(2)  It promotes tissue elements and strength;

(3)  It is very useful for infants, old people, emaciated persons, and for patients suffering from the diseases of the throat and lungs;

(4)   It promotes the corpulence of the body;

(5)   It helps in the healing of ulcers;

(6)   It promotes vital essence, hair and sharpness of the activities of sense organs;

(7)   It promotes longevity and vitality;

(8)   It cures poisoning; and

(9)   It alleviates *rluṅ* and *mkhris-pa*.

### Excessive Intake of Sweet Ingredients

Excessive intake of ingredients having sweet taste produces the following adverse effects :

(1)   It produces excess of *bad-kan* and fat;

(2)   It reduces the power of digestion;

(3)   It leads to obesity; and

(4)   It causes urinary disorders and obesity.

### Action of Ingredient Having Sour Taste

Intake of ingredients having sour taste produces the following actions :

(1)   It stimulates the power of digestion;

(2)   It is pleasing to the mind;

(3)   It scraps out sticky material from the body; and

(4)   It cures putrification and skin diseases.

### Excessive Intake of Sour Ingredients

Excessive intake of ingredients having sour taste produces the following adverse effects :

(1)   It obstructs the movement of *rluṅ*;

(2)   It produces a disease characterised by bleeding from different parts of the body;

(3) It causes looseness of the body-tissues;

(4) It causes cataract, giddiness, anemia and obstinate abdominal diseases including ascites; and

(5) It also causes erysipelas, itches, oedema, morbid thirst and infectious fever.

## Action of Ingredient Having Saline Taste

Intake of ingredients having saline taste produces the following effects :

(1) It cures stiffness in any part of the body;

(2) It removes obstruction to the channels of circulation;

(3) Its steam causes sweating; and

(4) It stimulates the power of digestion and makes food relishing.

## Excessive Intake of Saline Ingredients

Excessive intake of ingredients having saline taste produces the following adverse effects :

(1) It causes baldness, graying of the hair and wrinkles over the skin prematurely;

(2) It reduces strength; and

(3) It causes morbid thirst, obstinate skin diseases including leprosy, erysipelas and disease characterised by bleeding from different parts of the body.

## Action of Ingredient Having Bitter Taste

Intake of ingredients having bitter taste produces the following actions :

(1) It reduces excessive appetite by producing bad taste in the ingredients of food and drinks to which it is added;

(2)  It cures parasitic infestation, morbid thirst, poisoning, obstinate skin diseases including leprosy, fainting, infectious fever and aggravated *mkhris-pa*;

(3)  It dries up sticky material in the body, fat, bone-marrow, stool and urine; and

(4)  It promotes intellect, and cures breast-diseases and aphasia.

### Excessive Intake of Bitter Ingredients

Excessive intake of ingredients having bitter taste produces the following adverse actions :

(1)  It causes diminution of the tissue elements; and

(2)  It causes aggravation of *rluṅ* and *bad-kan*.

### Action of Ingredient Having Pungent Taste

Intake of ingredients having pungent taste produces the following actions :

(1)  It cures throat-diseases, constipation, obstinate skin diseases including leprosy and obstinate abdominal diseases including ascites;

(2)  It helps in healing ulcers;

(3)  It is digestive-stimulant and carminative;

(4)  It makes the food tasty;

(5)  It dries up fat and sticky material in the body; and

(6)  It cleanses the channels of circulation.

### Excessive Intake of Pungent Ingredients

Excessive intake of ingredients having pungent taste produces the following adverse effects :

(1)  It diminishes semen and strength;

(2) It causes contraction and trembling of the body; and

(3) It causes fainting and diseases of the lumber region, back, etc.

## *Action of Ingredient Having Astringent Taste*

Intake of ingredients having astringent taste produces the following actions :

(1) It dries up blood, *mkhris-pa*, fat and sticky material in the body;

(2) It helps in the healing of ulcers; and

(3) It promotes complexion of the skin.

## *Excessive Intake of Astringent Ingredients*

Excessive intake of ingredients having astringent taste produces the following adverse effects :

(1) It causes intestinal disorders;

(2) It causes constipation, obstruction to the passage of stool, flatulence, heart diseases, morbid thirst and obstruction to the channels of circulation.

Because of the specific nature of the conglomeration of the basic elements, there are certain exceptions to the above mentioned general rule. But in general, sweet ingredients alleviate *rluṅ* and *mkhris-pa* and aggravate *bad-kan*. Sour ingredients alleviate *bad-kan* and aggravate *mkhris-pa*. Saline ingredients alleviate *rluṅ* and *bad-kan*, and aggravate *mkhris-pa*. Bitter ingredients alleviate *mkhris-pa*, and aggravate *bad-kan* and *rluṅ*. Pungent ingredients alleviate *rluṅ* and *bad-kan*, and aggravate *mkhris-pa*. Astringent ingredients alleviate *mkhris-pa*, and aggravate *bad-kan* and *rluṅ*.

# Źu-rjes or Taste Emerging After Digestion

Different tastes described before are felt or perceived when a substance is placed over the tongue. But when the substance is digested and during the process of metabolism, because of the reactions of the enzymes, some other tastes develop which is called *źu-rjes*. These are of three types, viz., *mṅar* or sweet, *skyur* or sour, and *kha* or bitter. They are produced as follows :

(1) Sweet and sour ingredients generally become sweet in *źu-rjes*;

(2) Sour ingredients become same sour in *źu-rjes*; and

(3) Bitter, pungent and astringent ingredients become bitter in *źu-rjes*.

Ingredients having sweet *źu-rjes* alleviate *rluṅ* and *mkhris-pa*. Ingredients having sour *źu-rjes* alleviate *bad-kan* and *rluṅ*. Ingredients having bitter *źu-rjes* alleviate *mkhris-pa* and *bad-kan*.

There are exceptions to this general rule. It is possible that a different *źu-rjes* may emerge because of the specific conglomeration of the basic elements in the composition of a substance. In the texts, while describing drugs, ingredients of food, etc., mention of *źu-rjes* according to general rule is generally avoided unless it has any specific purpose to serve. But the *źu-rjes* which appear as exceptions to the general rule are specifically described.

## Yon-tan or Attributes

Apart from taste and *źu-rjes*, ingredients of drug and diet possess seventeen attributes as follows :

(1) *'Jam-pa* or smoothness;

(2) *Lci-ba* or heaviness;

(3) *Dro-ba* or heat;

(4) *Snum-pa* or unctuousness;

(5) *Brtan-pa* or stability;

These five attributes are related to the basic element *sa,* and they alleviate *rluṅ.*

(6)  *Graṅ-ba* or coldness;

(7)  *Brtul-ba* or softness;

(8)  *Bsil-ba* or coldness in excess;

(9)  *Mñen-pa* or tenderness;

(10)  *Sla-ba* or dullness;

(11)  *Skam-pa* or sliminess;

These six attributes (from nos. 6 to 11) are related to the basic element called *chu,* and they cause alleviation of *mkhris-pa.*

(12)  *Skya-ba* or non-sliminess;

(13)  *Tsha-ba* or heat in excess;

(14)  *Yaṅ-ba* or lightness;

(15)  *Rno-ba* or sharpness;

(16)  *Rtsub-pa* or ununctuousness; and

(17)  *G'yo-ba* or mobility.

These six attributes (from nos. 12 to 17) are related to the basic element called *me,* and they alleviate *bad-kan.*

These attributes of a substance are carefully examined to ascertain the therapeutic efficacy of a drug or food-ingredient for a particular type of *ñes-pa.*

## Nus-pa or Potency

Out of the seventeen attributes (*yon-tan*), eight become very prominent to produce therapeutic effects. These are called *nus-pa* or potency, and are as follows :

(1)  *Lci* or heaviness;

(2)  *Snum* or unctuousness;

(3)  *Bsil* or cold;

(4)  *Rtul-ba* or dullness;

(5)  *Yaṅ* or lightness;

(6)   *Rtsub* or ununctuousness;

(7)   *Tsha* or hot; and

(8)   *Rno-ba* or sharpness.

It will be seen from the above that these *nus-pas* are pairs having opposite effects, like heaviness and lightness, ununctuousness and unctuousness, cold and hot, and dullness and sharpness.

The first four of these potencies (nos. 1 to 4) alleviate *mkhris-pa*, and the remaining four (nos. 5 to 8) alleviate *bad-kan*. Lightness, ununctuousness and cold potencies aggravate *rluṅ*. Hot, sharpness and unctuousness aggravate *mkhris-pa*. Heaviness, unctuousness, cold and dullness cause aggravation of *bad-kan*.

Of these eight types of potencies, it is the hot and cold which are most important. Drugs having hot potency cure diseases caused by cold, and drugs having cold potency cure diseases caused by heat. It will be seen later that all the diseases are classified into two categories, viz., hot and cold.

It will be seen from the above that there is a close relationship between the basic elements composing a substance and its taste, *zu-rjes* (taste that is manifested after the digestion of the substance), attributes (*yon-tan*) and potencies (*nus-pa*). All these are also related to the three *ñes-pas*, viz., *rluṅ*, *mkhris-pa* and *bad-kan*. These *ñes-pas* are primarily responsible for the causation of various diseases. For the treatment of these diseases, therefore, drugs and diet having appropriate taste, *źu-rjes*, attribute and potency should be selected and administered.

## No-ba or Specific Action

In normal circumstances, it is the taste of a drug or diet which produces the therapeutic effect. At times, the effects of taste is surpassed by the effect of *żu-rjes* if it is not in harmony with the former. Similarly, the effect of *żu-rjes* is surpassed by the effect of the potency, if the latter is not in harmony with the former. At times, an absolutely new effect which is connected neither with taste or *żu-rjes* or attributes or potencies, is manifested because of specific nature of the conglomeration of the basic elements composing the substance, and reaction of the enzymes. This specific effect is called *ṅo-ba*.

The physician gets acquainted with these unique concepts of drug composition and drug action before he could successfully treat an ailment of the patient.

# 8

# Classification of Drugs and Food Articles

In Tibetan medicine, mostly natural products are used as medicine, food and drinks. Synthetic preparations are never used by the physicians. These ingredients are broadly classified into two categories, viz., those derived from living or animated sources (*sems-can*), and others derived from inanimate sources (*mi-sems-can*). The latter is further classified into two categories as follows :

(1) Natural products like metals, minerals, gems and precious stones; and

(2) Artificially prepared ingredients like certain types of salts.

Ingredients derived from animated or living sources are further divided into two groups, viz., (1) those derived from vegetable sources, and (2) those derived from animals. The vegetable kingdom is further sub-divided into four categories as follows :

(1) Trees having fruits, but with no apparent flowers;

(2) Trees having both fruits and flowers;

(3) Creepers; and

(4) Annual herbs.

The animal kingdom is further sub-divided in to four categories as follows :

(1) Mammals;

(2) Born of eggs;

(3)   Born out of heat and moistures; ;and
(4)   Born out of the earth.

Medicinal ingredients and ingredients used as food and drinks often overlap because there are many ingredients common to both. According to Tibetan medicine, food ingredients can be used as medicine and *vice versa*. The only significant difference between these two categories is that medicinal ingredients are dominated by *nus-pa* or potency and ingredients of food and drinks are dominated by *ro* or taste.

## Classification of Medicinal Ingredients

Medicinal ingredients are generally classified into eight categories as follows :

(1) *Precious Metals and Costly Stones*
This group includes gold, silver, copper, iron, turquoise, pearl, mother of pearl, conch-shell, coral and lapis lazuli.

(2) *Metals and Minerals*
This group includes magnetite, pyrites, natural cinnabar, red oxide of lead, zinc, Calcium sulphate, Calcium carbonate and alabastor, among others.

(3) *Medicinal Ingredients Collected from Earth*
This group includes golden sand, vermilion, Potassium nitrate, Potassium bicarbonate, sulphur, Copper sulphate and mineral-pitch, among others.

(4) *Herbal Medicines*
This group includes roots, trunks, stems, branches, pith, bark, exudate, leaves, flowers and fruits of different medicinal plants.

(5) *Exudates*

Exudates including gum-resins of different types of plants, and secretions of different animals are included in this group.

(6) *Decoctions*

Roots, tender branches, leaves, flowers and fruits used in the form of decoction are included in this group. Many recipes of decoctions which include camphor, red sandal-wood, bamboo-manna, saffron, small cardamom, big cardamom, cloves, cubeb, water-lilly, white cumin, black cumin, coriander, pomegranate, long pepper, black pepper, ginger, cinnamon, asafoetida, chebulic myrobalans, goose berry, mango, turmeric, liquorice, croton cassia, among others, are described under this group.

(7) *Medicinal Plants Used in Unboiled Form*

About one hundred plants which are used either in the form of juice or powder form without boiling are included in this group.

(8) *Animal Products*

Depending upon the part of the animal used in medicine, these are classified into thirteen sub-groups, viz., horns, bones, flesh, blood, bile, fat, brain, skin, nail, feather, urine, stool and whole animal.

Horns of rhinoceros, spotted deer, deer, ram, gazelle, wild yak and wild sheep are used in medicine.

Bones of tiger, cowrie-shell, pig, sheep, monkey and hooved animals among others, are used as medicine.

Flesh of the snake, vulture, pea-cock, iguana, otter, marmot, goat, wolf, pig, dog, ass, fox, bat, sparrow, mountain lizard and red wild duck, among others, are used in medicine.

Blood of deer, goat, wild yak, pig, ass and cock, among others is used in medicine.

Bile of different types of animals like cattle, elephant and bear is used in medicine.

The fat of snake, deer and pig among others, is used as medicine.

The brain of goat, sheep, rabbit and other wild animals, among others, is used in medicine.

The skin of snake, rhinoceros, bull and mouse is used in medicine.

The nail of crocodile, ass and horse (hooves), among others, is used in medicine.

The feather and hair of pea-cock, black-goose, owl, flying squirrel, baharal sheep and uncastrated goat is used in medicine.

Urine of human beings and cow is used in medicine.

The stool of vulture, pig, horse, rabbit, wolf, dog, cock, and pigeon is used in medicine.

Spanish fly, scorpion, caterpillar, snail, etc., are used in the form of the whole animal.

Many other plants, animals and metals including minerals and costly stones are used in Tibetan medicine. What is given above is only a brief enumeration.

## Classification of Food Ingredients

Ingredients used as food are classified into five categories as follows :

(1) *'Bru or Cereals and Pulses*
This group includes paddy, wheat, barley, buck-wheat, *Dolichos biflorus, Phaseolus radiatus, Lathyrus sativus, Lens culinaris, Sesamum indicum* and *Linum usitatissimum,* among others.

(2) *Sa or Meat of Animals*

Animals whose meat is used as food are further sub-
divided into eight groups as follows :

(i)   *Rko-ba'i sde or gallinaceous group.*

These are again subdivided into two groups, viz.,
those who scratch the earth with their claws or nails
for food, and those who dig the earth with the help of
their beaks for food.

Peacock, cock, partridge, crow, parrot, cuckoo-bird,
pigeon, magpie, chukor bird and sparrow, among
others, belong to this group.

(ii)  *Ri-dvags sde or small animals inhabiting thin forests*

This group includes deer, musk-deer, hog deer, wild
sheep, rabbit and antelope.

(iii) *Ri-dvags che ba'i sde or big animals inhabiting thick
forests*

This group includes nilgai, antelope, wild goat, wild
boar, wild buffalo, rhinoceros, leopard, wild ass and
wild yak.

(iv)  *Gcan gzan sde or pedatory wild beasts*

This group includes tiger, panther, bear, hyena, wolf,
wild cat, fox, jackal, monkey, etc.

(v)   *Rtsal mthus za ba'i sde or animals who eat by snatching
their food*

This group includes vulture, crow, eagle, kite and
sparrow.

(vi)  *Mi yis bdag byed sde or domesticated animals*

This includes hybrid cow, yak, camel, horse, ass,
cow, bullock, bull, goat, sheep, dog, pig, cock, cat,
etc.

(vii) *Khuṅ gnas sde or animals dwelling in burrows in the
earth*

This group includes marmot, hedge hot, frog, python,
iguana and scorpion.

(viii)  *Rlan la gnas pa'i sde or aquatic animals including those inhabiting marshy land*
This group includes crane, swan, pelican, gull, otter, fish, etc.

### (3) *Different Types of Fat*

This group includes fresh butter, ghee, cheese, sesame oil, mustard oil, bone-marrow, muscle fat, etc.

### (4) *No-ṅad or Aromatic Herbs Used in Uncooked Form*

This group includes onion, garlic, radish, turnip, mountain garlic, etc.

### (5) *Cooked Food*

This group includes different types of gruel, boiled rice, paddy pop, cooked barley, meat-soup and different other preparations of cereals, pulses and vegetables. Different types of spices used in food preparations are also included in this group.

## Classification of Drinks

Drinks are of three categories, viz., milk, water and alcoholic preparations.

### (1) *Milk and Milk Preparations*

In this group milk of cow, goat, sheep, female yak, mare, ass and different milk preparations like yoghurt, butter-milk, whey and cheese are included.

### (2) *Water*

This group includes different types of water like rain water collected directly from the sky, glacier water, stable water, water exposed to sun and air, polluted water, cold water, hot water and boiled but cooled water.

(3) *Alcoholic Drinks*

This group includes freshly prepared alcohol and old alcohol prepared from different types of cereals like wheat, rice and barley.

Properties of all the ingredients of medicine, food and drinks are described in Tibetan medical texts in great details. These ingredients are classified in different other ways by various Tibetan doctors. Masters and erudite scholars of Tibetan medicine like Sans-rgyas rgya-mtsho (1653 -1705 A.D.) and 'Jam-dpal rdo-rje (of Naiman who flourished in the beginning of 19th cent.) have provided illustrations of these ingredients in their illustrious works. Some of these ingredients are locally available in Tibet, and others are collected from the neighbouring countries.

The right hand of Medicine Buddha is adorned by a branch of the tree called *a-ru-ra (Terminalia chebula)*, and during religious ceremonies, the fruit of this tree is placed near Lord Buddha because of its auspicious nature. Medicinal ingredients are highly respected by physicians and common man alike as objects of auspiciousness. These are collected on auspicious days after performing religious rituals, and after collection and processing, are sanctified by holy incantations.

Different types of recipes in the form of juice, powder, pills, linctus, decoction, medicated ghee, medicated oils and alcoholic drinks are prepared from out of these ingredients. These represent rich store house of life-saving recipes for obstinate and otherwise incurable diseases, in addition to common diseases. Appropriately, and after scientific studies, if needed, these recipes can be used for curing the so called incurable diseases, and for mitigating the miseries of the suffering humanity. That these ingredients and recipes are successfully used for thousands of years against maladies is sufficient proof of their therapeutic efficacy.

## Grouping of Drugs as Recipes

These drugs, because of synergistic action and therapeutic utility are also categorised into several groups as follows :

(A) Group of Drugs for Alleviating Heat of the Body
  (1)  *Ga-bur* (camphor);
  (2)  *Tsan-dan dkar po* (white sandal wood);
  (3)  *Gi-waṅ* (solidified cattle bile);
  (4)  *Cu-gaṅ* (bamboo manna);
  (5)  *Gur-gum* (saffron); and
  (6)  *U-tpal sñon-po* (blue variety of water-lilly).

(B) Group of Drugs for Alleviating *Mkhris-pa*
  (1)  *Tig-ta (Swertia chirata)*;
  (2)  *Gser gyi me-tog (Momordica charantia)*;
  (3)  *Dug-ma-ñuṅ (Holarrhena antidysenterica)*;
  (4)  *Boṅ-ṅa dkar-po (Aconitum heterophyllum)*;
  (5)  *Rtsa-mkhris* (sow thistle);
  (6)  *G'ya'-ki-ma (Chrysosplenum nepalense)*;
  (7)  *Kyi-lca (Gentiana olivieri)*; and
  (8)  *Skyer-pa (Berberis aristata)*.

(C) Group of Drugs for Alleviating *Rluṅ*
  (1)  *Dza-ti (Myristica fragnace)*;
  (2)  *Bu-ram* (jaggery); and
  (3)  *Rus* (bones of different animals).

(D) Group of Drugs for Alleviating *Bad-kan* and *Rluṅ*
  (1)  *Sman-ga* (dried rhizome of *Zingiber officinale*);
  (2)  *Sga-skya* (fresh rhizome of *Zingiber officinale*);
  (3)  *Siṅ-kun (Ferula foetida)*;
  (4)  *Kha-ru-tsha* (black salt); and
  (5)  *Btson-sgog (Allium cepa)*.

In addition to the above, several other groups of drugs are described in Tibetan works for the following :

(1)    To cure blood diseases;

(2)    To cure infectious diseases;

(3)    To cure lung diseases;

(4)    To cure aggravated *rluṅ* associated with fever;

(5)    To cure aggravated *bad-kan* associated with fever;

(6)    To cure aggravated *bad-kan* associated with cold;

(7)    To cure lymph disorders;

(8)    To cure parasitic infestations;

(9)    To cure diarrhoea; and

(10)   To cure urinary disorders.

The method of preparing a recipe by the permutation and combination of these and such other ingredients for multi-dimensional and multi-faceted therapeutic effects is also elaborated in Tibetan texts.

# 9

# Preventive Medicine and Positive Health

Treatment of diseases is to be attempted when these are already manifested because of the person's ignorance or deliberate violation of the health-rules. But Tibetan medicine emphasises upon the prevention of diseases and maintenance as well as promotion of positive health for which several dos and don'ts, and conducts are prescribed for different parts of the day and night and for different seasons of the year.

## Rgyun Spyod or Conducts for the Day

Every day a person should observe proper conduct in worldly affairs for happiness and long span of life. In addition, he should observe some sacred regimens to give him happiness in the present life and in the life after death. The worldly conducts are as follows :

(1) One should always wear gems and talismans containing sacred incantations;

(2) One should use appropriate food and regimens in accordance with his own profession and seasons;

(3) One should avoid ten sinful acts through his body, speech and mind;

(4) One should not torture the sense organs like tongue, etc., nor should these senses be appeased in excess;

(5) One should avoid sailing in an undependable boat,

and riding over violent or dangerous animals and vehicles;

(6) One should avoid travelling through the places where animals and human beings are killed, and should not enter into places having a big fire;

(7) One should avoid walking over deep crevices, and climbing to the top of big trees;

(8) One should reside or seat in a place after proper examination;

(9) If one has to move out of the home for any important work at night, then he should be well equipped with security measures and accompanied by friends;

(10) One should avoid remaining awake at night. If for emergent reasons, one has to remain awake at night, then he should observe fast, and in the next day, should sleep for half the period of remaining awake at previous night;

(11) One should not sleep normally during the day time. However, persons who are intoxicated, emaciated, afflicted with grief, exposed to physical exercise, indulging in long speech, very old, very young and fearful may sleep during the day time. In summer, all people may sleep during day time;

(12) If one does not get sleep during night time, he should take milk, yoghurt (curd), alcohol, meat soup, etc. His head should be massaged with oil and oil should be poured into his ears;

(13) In case of excessive sleep, one should keep fast and have sexual intercourse;

(14) One should avoid sex relationship in the genital organs of animals, with a woman married to another person, a woman who is not beautiful to look at, with a pregnant woman, with a woman who does not like sex, who is weak, who gets pain during sexual

intercourse, with a woman during her period of menstruation, and with a woman who does not want to be a sex partner;

(15) In winter, a person can have sexual intercourse very frequently. During autumn and in spring seasons, one should have sexual intercourse for not more than once in two days. During the rainy season and summer, one should have sexual intercourse for not more than once in a fortnight;

(16) For the prevention of aging process and fatigue, and for the alleviation of *rluṅ*, oil massage should be done every day over the whole body, specially over the head and feet. Oil should be poured into the ears habitually;

(17) One should perform exercise (not exceeding one's own strength) which causes lightness of the body, reduces fat, makes the body muscular, stimulates the power of digestion, makes the body sturdy, and enhances the ability of a person to perform his work;

(18) One should apply *dril-phyi* or unction over his body to reduce excess of fat, promote lustre of the skin and give rise to excellent stability of the limbs;

(19) One should take bath daily. It stimulates sex-desire, and promotes the power of digestion, strength, longevity and vital essence. It cures itching, excessive perspiration, foul smell, laziness, thirst and burning sensation in the body;

(20) One should apply collyrium in the eyes regularly once in every seven days to protect and promote eye-sight;

(21) One should not enjoy good things by himself alone. The enjoyable things should be equally shared with others;

(22) One should eternally and closely strive not to cast himself upon miseries. He should follow the religious prescriptions and prohibitions;

(23) One should keep to his words (promise), and give appropriate replies to queries;

(24) One should shun bad actions, should not be afraid of performing good actions even if that makes him to face several difficult situations;

(25) Before undertaking any activities, one should always examine the pros and cons;

(26) Do not accept anything as truth because of here say. Accept it only after proper examination;

(27) One should examine all pros and cons, and thereafter, give a reply in brief which should be meaningful and to the point;

(28) One should not listen to irrelevant talks and should not disclose his secrets to others;

(29) To a friend one should not be deceitful, and should talk to him straightforwardly;

(30) One should perform controlled and disciplined action which endows friendship and happiness instantaneously;

(31) Never allow the enemy to go scot-free, choose appropriate and far-sighted means to subdue him;

(32) Attendants should be looked with love. With far-sight think of their sincere work exhibited earlier and forgive for their temporary mistakes;

(33) Be respectful to mother, father and senior relatives in the family;

(34) Be amiable and friendly to your countrymen and enjoy their companionship;

(35) Be thrifty in business, and at times and need, donate in charity liberally;

(36) If a mistake is committed knowingly or unknowingly, accept it gracefully. If one is victorious, then he should draw limited satisfaction and should not be overexcited because of victory;

(37) One should not exhibit ego for his scholarship. A wealthy person should be satisfied with his possession, and should not hanker after more and more of wealth;

(38) One should not humiliate sub-ordinates, and should not be jealous of others who are holding higher ranks;

(39) One should not have close relationship with bad people, and should not have enmity with priests and saints;

(40) One should not steal other's wealth and possession, and should avoid taking oath to retaliate others;

(41) To achieve one's objectives in life, one should take firm steps to avoid regrets; and

(42) With far-sighted mental power, one should perform his duties appropriately and in time.

Apart from these worldly codes of conduct, a person should perform his religious duties to be healthy and happy.

## Religious and Sacred Duties

Every living creature desires happiness for which efforts should be directed towards religion. Otherwise, their very desire for happiness becomes the cause of unhappiness. Therefore, one should make efforts to attend to religious duties with devotion and friendly feelings for all living creatures. Through body, speech and mind one should shun ten categories of sinful acts which are as follows :

(1) *Srog-gcod* or violence, i.e. causing harm to or killing animals;

(2)   *Rku* or stealing other's possessions;
(3)   *Long-por g'yem-pa* or sexual misconduct;
(4)   *Rdzun* or making false statements;
(5)   *Nag-'khyal* or idle gossip;
(6)   *Tshig-rtsub* or abusive speech;
(7)   *Dbyen-sbyor* or slanderous speech;
(8)   *Brabs-sems* or jealousy;
(9)   *Gnod-sems* or malice towards others; and
(10)  *Lta-ba phyin-ci-log* or misguided views.

The religious practice referred to above does not mean the practice of Buddhism alone. A person is free to practice the religion of his own faith.

## Regimens for Different Seasons

Apart from the code of conduct, both worldly and religious, a person should adopt appropriate regimens during different seasons for the preservations and promotion of positive health and prevention of diseases. The *ñes-pas* naturally undergo the process of accumulation and aggravation during different seasons. If proper care is taken through regimens, then instead of spreading to other parts of the body for causing diseases, they will automatically get alleviated.

There are six different seasons as follows :
(1)   *Dgun-stod* or early part of the winter;
(2)   *Dgun-smad* or the later part of the winter;
(3)   *Dpyid* or spring;
(4)   *So-ga* or summer;
(5)   *Dbyar* or rainy season; and
(6)   *Ston* or autumn.

## Regimens for Early Part of Winter

Because of the cold, in the early winter the hair-follicles get obstructed, and the heat inside the body becomes stronger. During this season, if the food is consumed in less quantity, then the tissue elements of the body get burnt and diminished. Therefore, during this period, a person should consume more of food, particularly those containing sweet, sour and saline ingredients.

During this period, nights are long, and a person becomes very hungry when he gets up from the bed in the morning. Because of this, the tissue elements may also get diminished. Therefore, a person should take heavy snack during break-fast.

Massage with the help of sesame oil is very useful to alleviate *rluṅ* which gets aggravated normally during this period. One should take heavy and nourishing food like the meat and meat-soup of different animals. Fomentation therapy, and exposure to the hot rays of the sun and fire are very useful during this period. One should preferably reside inside a under-ground house having thick walls.

## Regimens for the Later Part of Winter

The later part of the winter is very cold, and all the regimens for the early part of the winter should also be followed during this period with added care.

## Regimens for Spring

In the later of the winter, *bad-kan* gets accumulated because of the cold. During spring, because of the exposure to the heat of the sun, *bad-kan* gets aggravated. As a result of this, the power of digestion and metabolism gets suppressed. Therefore, during this period, a person should consume more of pungent, bitter and astringent ingredients. In addition, he should take old-barley, meat of animals inhabiting in arid zone, honey, boiled water and decoction of ginger in liberal quantities. He should resort to physical exercise and unction regularly. One should sit in the sun-shade in a fragrant and pleasing park during the day time.

## Regimens for Summer

The hot rays of the sun during the summer season reduces the strength of a person. Therefore, one should consume more of sweet and unctuous ingredients having cooling effect. One should avoid food ingredients having saline, pungent and sour tastes. One should take frequent bath in cold water, and take alcoholic drinks well diluted with cold water. One should wear very thin clothes and reside in a cooling house. During the day time, one should sit in the shade of trees enjoying the pleasant aroma of the flowering trees.

## Regimens of Rainy Season

During the rainy season, the sky remains cloudy for the most part, and because of rains, there is great deal of humidity in the atmosphere. The wind becomes cold but because of the rains, heat comes out of the earth. The water becomes dirty which suppresses the power of digestion. Therefore, one should take such food and drinks which stimulate the power of digestion like those having sweet, sour and saline tastes. One should take light and unctuous food, and drink alcohol prepared of cereals growing the arid zone. One should reside in the top floor of the house which is free from cold wind and humidity.

## Regimens for Autumn

During this season, the hot rays of the sun cause aggravation of *mkhris-pa*. For its alleviation, one should take food and drinks ingredients of which are sweet, bitter and astringent in taste. One should use clothes which are smeared with aromatic ingredients like camphor and sandal-wood paste or oils. The house where one stays should also be sprinkled with these aromatic ingredients.

To summarize, during the rainy season and winters, one should take food and drinks which are hot in potency; in the spring, one should take food and drinks which are unctuous; and in the summer as well as autumn, one should take cooling things.

During the rainy season and winters, ingredients having sweet, sour and saline tastes should be used; during spring season, ingredients having pungent, bitter and astringent tastes should be used; and during the autumn season, sweet, bitter and astringent ingredients should be used.

In the autumn season, purgation therapy is useful; in the spring season, emetic therapy is useful; and in the rainy season, oleating type of medicated enema is useful.

What is described above is only an outline of the regimens to be followed during different seasons. A physician can make necessary changes in the diet, etc., depending upon the actual requirements of a person. In the texts of Tibetan medicine, all these regimens are described in great detail.

Following these codes of conduct and regimens for different seasons, a person leads a physically, mentally and spiritually healthy and happy life.

# 10

# Diseases and Their Classification

The etiology of all diseases is broadly classified into two categories as follows :
(1) *Rgyu* or primary cause; and
(2) *Rkyen* or secondary cause.

The primary causes of the disease are of two types, viz., *riṅ-rgyu* or distant cause, and *ñe-rgyu* or nearby cause. *Ma-rig* or ignorance is the distant primary cause of all the diseases. This gives rise to *'dod-chags* or passion, *źe-ldaṅ* or anger, and *gti-mug* or illusion. From these three factors, three morbid causing factors, viz., *rluṅ, mkhris-pa* and *bad-kan* take origin respectively which constitute the *ñe-rgyu* or nearby causes of all diseases. These three factors taken together are called *ñes-pa*. They remain in a state of equilibrium in a healthy person. Any disturbance in their equilibrium gives rise to diseases and death. Such disturbances are caused by a group of factors called *rkyen* or secondary causative factors.

The secondary causative factors are classified into three categories as follows :
(1) *Dus* or temporal factors;
(2) *Dbaṅ-po* or sensory factors; and
(3) *Spyod-lam* or regimens including activities.

*Dus* or temporal factors are the variations of temperature and humidity in different seasons which cause accumulation, aggravation and spreading of the *ñes-pas*. Such morbidities normally take place within limits and the body has the inbuilt power to overcome such minor changes. By following prescribed regimens, these aggravated *ñes-pas* get automatically alleviated, and do not cause a disease.

Non-utilisation, excessive utilisation and wrong utilisation of the sense faculties cause aggravation of these *ñes-pas* to cause diseases.

Similarly, the *spyod-lam* or activities including conduct through the body, mind and speech, if performed inappropriately cause aggravation of these *ñes-pas* leading to diseases.

Apart from the endogenous factors described above, several exogenous factors like affliction by evil spirits, poisons and weapons also cause diseases. Administration of contradictory therapies also causes diseases by aggravating the *ñes-pas*.

Diseases, according to Tibetan medicine, are classified in different ways. On the basis of the causative factors, these are of three types as follows :

(1) Those caused by the aggravation or vitiation of the three *ñes-pas* because of bad food, drinks, conducts and regimens inappropriate to different seasons;

(2) Those caused by the sinful acts of the past life and even earlier part of the present span of life; and

(3) Those caused by the combination of both the first and second categories of causative factors described above.

On the basis of the place of manifestation, diseases are classified into five categories as follows :

(1) Diseases of males;

(2) Female diseases;

(3) Diseases of children;

(4) Diseases of old people; and

(5) Diseases common to all the ages and sex.

Male diseases are of 17 varieties. Female diseases are of 14 varieties. Children diseases are of 24 varieties. Diseases of old people are caused by the diminution of the basic elements composing the body of the individual. Diseases common to all ages are as follows :

(1) Diseases caused by *rluṅ* are of 42 varieties;

(2) Diseases cause by *mkhris-pa* are of 26 varieties;

(3) Diseases caused by *bad-kan* are of 33 varieties;

(4) Diseases according to predominant causative factors, viz., aggravation and diminution of the *ñes-pas* are of 74 categories;

(5) Obstinate and serious diseases are of 27 varieties;

(6) Diseases afflicting the mind are of two types;

(7) Diseases located in the head and neck are of 18 varieties;

(8) Diseases located in the solid and hollow visceras are of 19 varieties;

(9) Diseases located in the lower parts of the body are of 5 varieties;

(10) Diseases located in the exterior of the body are of 20 varieties;

(11) Diseases pervading the entire body are of 37 varieties;

(12) Internal diseases are of 48 varieties;

(13) Ulcers are of 15 varieties;

(14) Fevers are of 19 varieties; and

(15) Other miscellaneous diseases are of 19 varieties.

To sum up, diseases caused by *ñes-pas* are of 101 varieties (*rluṅ*=42, *mkhris-pa*=26, and *bad-kan* = 33) —vide item nos. 1 to 3 above. On the basis of predominance and diminution of causative factors, diseases are of 101 varieties—vide item nos. 4 and 5 above. Diseases of the mind and body are of 101 varieties—vide item nos. 6 to 11 above. Based on varieties, diseases are of 101 varieties—vide item nos. 12 to 15 above. Thus, in total, diseases are classified into 404 varieties.

The above mentioned 404 varieties of diseases are further subdivided into four categories each as follows :

(1) Diseases leading to death even if properly treated;

(2) Diseases caused by the affliction of evil spirits which can be treated both by medicines and religious rituals;

(3) Diseases which get cured by proper treatment, but if proper treatment is not provided they cause death; and

(4) Minor diseases which get cured of their own even without any treatment.

Keeping the above subdivisions in view, all the 404 types of diseases can be subdivided into 1616 subvarieties. All these varieties and subvarieties can be broadly grouped into two broad categories, viz., hot diseases and cold diseases.

## Examination of Diseases

The physician, before attempting treatment, examines both the diseases and the patient. Diseases are examined with reference to the following aspects :

(1) Etiology which includes both *rgyu* (the primary causative factors) and *rkyen* (the secondary causative factors);

(2) Pre-monitory signs and symptoms (*snar-tshul*);

(3) Actual signs and symptoms of the disease (*nad-rtags*); and

(4) Pathogenic process (*dkyel-gyur*) with reference to number (*rnam-grans*), differential diagnosis (*brtag-pa*), predominance of one or other causative factors (*gtso-bo*) and strength of the diseases (*stobs*).

With the above mentioned methods of examination, the physician arrives at the diagnosis of the disease. Some of these common diseases are given a name. There are so many diseases afflicting human beings that giving a name for each one of them in a text becomes well nay impossible. The physician, therefore, is advised not to give too much importance to these names of the diseases. The unnamed diseases are to be treated by the physician on the basis of the *ñes-pas, lus-zuṅs* (tissue elements) and *dri-mas* (waste products) involved in their pathogenesis. The common diseases which are named and described with reference to their etiology, premonitory signs and symptoms, actual signs and symptoms, pathogenesis and treatment will be described hereafter.

## Common Diseases Described in Medical Texts

With reference to diagnosis and treatment, the following diseases are described in the classical texts of Tibetan medicine :

(1)   Diseases caused by *rluṅ* in general;
(2)   Diseases caused by *mkhris-pa* in general;
(3)   Diseases caused by *bad-kan* in general;
(4)   *Ma-źu-ba* or suppression of the power of digestion;
(5)   *Skran-nad* or phantom tumour;
(6)   *Skya-bab* or anemia;
(7)   *'Or-nad* or oedema;
(8)   *Dmu-chu* or ascites;
(9)   *Zas-byed* or tuberculosis;
(10)  *Tshad-pa* or fever of different types;
(11)  *Mgo-nad* or head diseases;
(12)  *Mig-nad* or eye diseases;
(13)  *Rna-ba'i nad* or ear diseases;
(14)  *Sna-nad* or nose diseases;
(15)  *Kha-nad* or mouth diseases;
(16)  *Lba-ba* or goiter;
(17)  *Sñiṅ-nad* or heart diseases;

(18)   *Glo-nad* or lungs diseases;

(19)   *Mchin-nad* or liver diseases;

(20)   *Mcher-nad* or spleen diseases;

(21)   *Mkhal-nad* or kidney diseases;

(22)   *Pho-ba'i nad* or stomach diseases;

(23)   *Rgyu-ma'i nad* or diseases of the small intestine;

(24)   *Loṅ-nad* or diseases of the large intestine;

(25)   *Pho-mtshan gyi nad* or diseases of male genital organs;

(26)   *Mo-tshan gyi nad* or diseases of female genital organs,

(27)   *Skad-'gags* or hoarseness of voice;

(28)   *Yi-ga 'chus-pa* or anorexia;

(29)   *Skom-nad* or morbid thirst;

(30)   *Skyigs-bu'i nad* or  hic-cup;

(31)   *Dbugs-mi bde-ba* or asthma;

(32)   *Glan-thabs* or colic pain;

(33)   *Srin-nad* or worm-infestation specially intestinal parasites;

(34)   *Skyugs-pa'i nad* or vomiting;

(35)   *'Khru-ba'i nad* or diarrhoea;

(36)   *Dri-ma 'gags-pa* or constipation;

(37)   *Chu-'gags* or urinary obstruction;

(38)   *Gcin-sñi-ba'i nad* or obstinate urinary disorders including diabetes;

(39)   *Tshad-pa'i 'khru-ba* or fever associated with diarrhoea;

(40)   *Dreg-nad* or gout;

(41)   *Grum-bu'i nad* or different forms of arthritis;

(42)   *Chu-ser gyi nad* or rheumatism;

(43)   *Rtsa-dkar gyi nad* or diseases characterised by whiteness of the veins;

(44)   *Lpag-pa'i nad* or skin diseases;

(45)   *Phran-bu'i nad* or minor diseases;

(46)   *Lhan-skyes rma* or endogenous ulcers;

(47)   *'Bras* or cervical adenitis;

(48) *Gzan-'brum* or piles;

(49) *Me-dbal* or erysipelas;

(50) *Sur-ya'i nad* or herpes;

(51) *Rmen-bu* or tumours;

(52) *Rlig-rlugs* or scrotal tumour including hernia and hydrocele;

(53) *Rkan-bam gyi nad* or filariasis (elephantiasis);

(54) *Mtshan-bar rdol-ba* or fistula-in-ano;

(55) *Byis-pa'i nad* or children diseases in general;

(56) *Byis-pa'i gdon* or children diseases caused by the affliction of evil spirits;

(57) *Mo-nad gtso-bo* or important female diseases in general;

(58) *Mo-nad bye-brag* or female diseases in special;

(59) *Mo-nad phal-pa* or female diseases of secondary importance;

(60) *'Byun-po'i gdon* or affliction by evil spirits;

(61) *Smyo-byed kyi gdon* or insanity caused by evil spirits;

(62) *Brjed-byed kyi nad* or epilepsy;

(63) *Gza'i gdon-nad* or affliction by evil demons;

(64) *Gdug-pa klu'i gdon* or affliction by evil serpent-demons;

(65) *Rma spyi* or ulcers in general;

(66) *Mgo-ba'i rma* or ulcers in the head;

(67) *Ske'i rma* or ulcers in the neck;

(68) *Byan-khog stod smad rma* or ulcers in the trunk;

(69) *Yan-lag gi rma* or ulcers in the limbs;

(70) *Sbyar-pa'i dug* or ailments caused by artificially prepared poisons;

(71) *Gyur-ba'i dug* or ailments caused by substances which become poisonous by exposure to sun, wind, etc.;

(72) *Rgyu-ba dan mi-rgyu-ba'i dug* or ailments caused by poisons of animate and inanimate origin;

(73) *Rgyas-pa gso-ba bcud-len* or rejuvenating therapies for the treatment of geriatric ailments;

(74)   *Ro-tsa-bar bya* or aphrodisiac therapies for impotency;
       and

(75)   *Bu-med-pa btsal-ba* or female sterility.

One should not carry the impression that these are the only diseases known to Tibetan physicians. These are described only by way of illustration with special reference to their diagnosis and treatment. Following the same line, other diseases which the physician comes across should be treated. Some of the so called modern diseases like AIDS and cancer can also be treated by the Tibetan physician with great success.

# 11

# Diagnostic Methods

A patient according to Tibetan medicine, is examined in three different ways, viz., (1) *blta* or observation, (2) *reg-pa* or palpation, and (3) *dri-ba* or interrogation. By interrogation, information regarding the causative factors of the disease like food, drinks and conduct could be ascertained. The subjective symptoms from which the patient is suffering could also be ascertained by this method. This will help the physician to determine the *ñes-pa* which is responsible for the causation of the disease, and the exact nature of the disease.

The tongue and the urine are examined by *blta* or observation. Reddishness, dryness and roughness of the tongue indicate the aggravation of *rluṅ*. If the tongue is covered with thick and yellowish material, then *mkhris-pa* is aggravated. If the tongue is gray, thick, lustreless and smooth, then it is indicative of the aggravation of *bad-kan*. Urine examination provides authentic data regarding the exact nature and prognosis of the disease.

Examination of the pulse is the most important diagnostic tool which is performed by *reg-pa* or palpation.

## Pulse Examination

To diagnose a disease correctly in order to select the most appropriate therapy, and to predict the prognosis of the ailment by the examination of the pulse of the patient or even of his close relatives is one of the significant features of Tibetan medicine. The expertise in this field develops in different stages. Ordinary physicians can determine the aggravation of either *rluṅ* or *mkhris pa* or *bad-kan* from the pulse examination, and decide upon the mode of treatment required by the patient. An experienced physician can find out the morbidity in the solid and hollow visceras (vital organs) in the patient to suggest the exact therapeutic measures required by him. An expert physician dedicated to the practice of the mantra of Bhaiṣajya-guru (Medicine Buddha) can diagnose even the ailments of the close relatives like husband, wife, son, daughter, father and mother by examining the pulse of another person. Apart from the physical ailments, the physician can also ascertain the conditions of the mind and spirit of the patient through pulse examination.

Unnatural or stimulating food, drinks and regimens may interfere with the pulse examination. Therefore, the patient should not take heavy food, alcoholic drinks and such other stimulating and heavy ingredients in the night prior to the examination of pulse. He should have slept well (unless he is suffering from insomnia) and should not indulge in sexual intercourse during the night before the examination of pulse. Since pulse examination needs a lot of concentration of mind, the physician should also avoid such heavy food, drinks and sexual intercourse.

The best time for the examination of pulse is the early morning after the patient has visited toilet and when in a relaxed mood and in empty stomach. Of course, pulse can be examined any time in an emergency. But it should be ensured that the food and drinks consumed by the patient earlier are already digested. In the case of female patients, pulse examination should be avoided during their menstrual period because of the hormonal disturbance associated with it. But if the patient has any gyenic ailment, pulse examination can be done even during this period.

Generally, pulse is examined over the radial artery in the hand. Tibetan doctors examine the pulse of both the hands of the patient. In the female patients, the right hand pulse is examined first followed by the left hand. In the case of male patients, the pulse of the left hand is examined first followed by the right hand. During pulse examination, the patient sits in front of the physician. The physician, with the help of his palm supports the hand of the patient at the elbow joint. With his right hand, he examines the pulse of the left hand of the patient, and with his left hand he examines the pulse of the right hand of the patient. Adept physicians even examine the pulse of both the hands simultaneously.

Over the radial artery which is located below the thumb, the physician puts three of his fingers, namely the index, middle and ring fingers simultaneously and applies uniform pressure. The hand of the patient should be slightly bent at the wrist joint so that the lines below the thumb are clearly visible. Below the prominent line, the space equal to the size of the thumb of the patient should be left out, and thereafter, the index finger should be placed followed by the remaining fingers in such a way that the fingers of the physician should be closed to each other, but should not touch each other. With his three fingers, the physician places uniform pressure over the artery. Since the space below the index finger is bony, and the space below the ring finger is fleshy, for uniformity of the pressure on the artery, the index finger should be lightly pressed, the middle finger should be pressed slightly more, and the ring finger should be pressed much more. This technique is important, and is perfected through a long practice.

Apart from the rate, rythm, volume and tension, the Tibetan physician is more concerned with how and where he feels the pulsation. If the pulse gives an empty feeling, and there are missing beats, then this indicates aggravation of *rluṅ*. Aggravation of *mkhris-pa* is indicated by quick, spreading and subtle pulse. If *bad-kan* is aggravated, then the physician feels as if the artery is sunk to the bottom, and it is weak as well as slow.

The physician, with concentration of mind, repeatedly examines the pulse by withdrawing the pressure and again pressing the radial artery. He then examines where the pulsation is felt. For this purpose, the finger tips of the physician are divided into two parts—the upper or external part and the lower or internal part. The feeling of the pulse in the former part indicates morbidities in the solid visceras, and the feeling in the latter indicates the morbidities in the hollow visceras.

In male patients, while examining the pulse of his left hand, the feeling (pulsation) obtained by the physician, while examining through the fingers of his right hand, indicates morbidities as under :

(1)  The feeling of pulsation in the upper part of the index finger indicates morbidity in the heart;

(2)  The feeling of pulsation in the lower part of the index finger indicates the morbidity in the small intestine;

(3)  The feeling of pulsation in the upper part of the middle finger indicates the morbidity in the spleen;

(4)  The feeling of pulsation in the lower part of the middle finger indicates morbidity in the stomach;

(5)  The feeling of pulsation in the upper part of the ring finger indicates morbidity in the left kidney; and

(6)  The feeling of pulsation in the lower part of the ring finger indicates morbidity in the *bsam se'u* (genital organs).

In male patients, while examining the pulse of his right hand, the feeling (pulsation) obtained by the physician, while examining through the fingers of his left hand indicates morbidities as under :

(1) The feeling of pulsation in the upper part of the index finger indicates morbidity in the lungs;

(2) The feeling of pulsation in the lower part of the index finger indicates morbidities in the large intestine;

(3) The feeling of pulsation in the upper part of the middle finger indicates morbidity in the liver;

(4) The feeling of pulsation in the lower part of the middle finger indicates morbidities in the gall-bladder;

(5) The feeling of pulsation in the upper part of the ring finger indicates morbidities in the right kidney; and

(6) The feeling of pulsation in the lower part of the ring finger indicates morbidities in the urinary bladder.

In female patients, while examining the pulse of her right hand, the feeling (pulsation) obtained by the physician, while examining through the fingers of his left hand indicates morbidities as under :

(1) The feeling of pulsation in the upper part of the index finger indicates morbidities in the heart; and

(2) The feeling of pulsation in the lower part of the index finger indicates morbidities in the small intestine.

The feelings in the remaining fingers indicate similar morbidities as in the case of male patients.

In female patients, while examining the pulse of her left hand, the feeling (pulsation) obtained by the physician, while examining with the fingers of his right hand indicates morbidities as under :

(1) The feeling of pulsation in the upper part of the index finger indicates morbidities in the lungs; and

(2) The feeling of pulsation in the lower part of the index finger indicates morbidities in the large intestine.

The feelings in the remaining fingers indicate similar morbidities as in the case of male patients.

What is described above is just an outline of the method followed by Tibetan physicians for examining the pulse of a patient. In actual practice, pulse examination by the physicians of Tibetan medicine is very profound and subtle.

## Urine Examination

Next to pulse, urine is perhaps the most important diagnostic tool for the diagnosis of the disease for determining the exact treatment required by the patient, and for eliciting information regarding the prognosis of the disease. Urine is one of the three important waste products which is regularly excreted from the body. Along with the aqueous material, urine carries many soluble and insoluble ingredients from the blood and the urinary tract, thereby imparting specific colour, odour, turbidity, etc. to it. The other two important waste products which are regularly excreted from the body are the sweat and the stool, and they considerably influence the nature of the urine during different parts of the day and night, and during different seasons. These normal physiological changes are always to be kept in view while examining urine for the diagnostic purpose, and for arriving at the prognosis of the disease.

Depending upon the seasonal effects, during different parts of the day, the colour of the normal urine varies from absolute transparency to yellowishness. It has characteristic urinous odour and free from any sediment.

The food, drinks and conduct of the patient during the previous night may considerably affect the physical and chemical nature of the urine. In order to prevent such superimposed characteristics which may interfere in the exact diagnosis, the patient should avoid taking any heavy food, alcohol, etc., and should refrain from sexual intercourse. Urine examination of women during their menstruation should be avoided, and while collecting urine for examination, it should be ensured that the physiological and pathological secretions of the nearby genital tract does not get mixed up with the urine.

For examination, urine should be collected during the early morning, and the examination should be carried out as early as possible before any significant change, both physical and chemical, takes place in it. Both in males and females, the first and the last parts of the urine-flow should be rejected, and the urine of the middle part only should be collected for examination. The container or bottle to be used for containing urine should be of glass. It should be free from any greasy material or chemical used for washing it. It should be well capped to prevent dust and wind.

For actual examination, urine should be poured into a porcelain or glass beaker which is also free from greasy material and traces of the chemical used for its washing.

The urine examination is carried out in three different stages as follows:

(1) When it is fresh and warm;
(2) During the process of its becoming cold; and
(3) After it has become cold.

Apart from colour, odour, vapour (which emanates from the surface of the urine when it is exposed to air), turbidity (caused by suspended material in the urine) and sediments (which settle down at the bottom of the collecting bottle), urine is specially examined with reference to the bubbles which emanate when it is stirred with the help of a bundle of fine sticks. About five or six slender sticks having flat bottom are loosely tied with a thread at the middle portion, and the urine is stirred with it. The nature of the bubble, the way these appear and disappear are examined.

Diseases are caused by the aggravation or vitiation of three *ñes-pas*, viz., *rluṅ*, *mkhris-pa* and *bad-kan*, among others and their vitiation produces some characteristic changes in the urine. Thus, by urine examination, the physician can ascertain the condition of these *ñes-pas* which enables him to correctly diagnose the disease, and predict the prognosis.

If *rluṅ* is aggravated, the urine becomes brownish gray in colour and slightly odorous. Moderate quantity of steam comes out of it which disappears quickly. The urine is less turbid. When stirred, large size bubbles of bluish white colour appear which remain for sometime and then disappear. The sediments are of fibrous nature, and they are so light that often they remain suspended throughout the entire urine.

If *mkhris-pa* is aggravated, the colour of the urine becomes yellow or dark-red, and strong pungent or putrid smell comes out of it. The urine produces profuse quantity of steam which continues to emanate for a long time. The urine is turbid. When stirred, bubbles of small size and yellowish colour appear in large quantity, and they disappear quickly. Large quantity of sediment appear in this type of urine.

If there is aggravation of *bad-kan*, then the urine becomes milky white in colour. There is less of odour, and less of steam emanate from it. It is turbid in nature. When stirred, bubbles of small size and close to each other appear in large quantity. These bubbles do not disappear even after stirring is over for a long time.

The urine exhibit different other characteristic features to indicate the simultaneous vitiation of two or all the three of these *ñes-pas*. Some of these characteristic features even indicate the exact nature of the disease and its prognosis. Such detailed study of the urine needs profound theoretical knowledge and practical experience under the supervision of an expert Master.

# 12

# Principles of Treatment

Therapies and drugs of Tibetan medicine are generally classified into two categories, viz., *stobs-skyed* or nourishing therapy which promotes strength, and *nams-dmad* or lightening therapy which causes depletion of the tissue elements.

## Nourishing Therapy

Nourishing therapy is indicated when *rluṅ* is aggravated, for a person who is emaciated of tissue elements because of malnutrition, excessive physical work, grief, penance and excessive indulgence in sex, for a pregnant woman, if there is excessive bleeding during parturition, in phthisis, for a person of old age, if there is insomnia, and in summer season.

Food ingredients like mutton, jaggery, sugar, ghee, butter, milk, yoghurt and alcohol are nourishing by nature. Recipes of medicated ghee are nourishing. Oleating type of medicated enema, bath and body-massage are also nourishing in nature. Similarly sound sleep, leisurely living and happiness of mind cause nourishment of the body.

Nourishing therapy promotes the immunitary system of the body, strength and power to overcome the attacks of diseases. But if nourishing therapy is used in excess, this may give rise to diseases like obesity, abscess, lymphadenitis, cough, obstinate urinary diseases including diabetes mellitus, and aggravation of *bad-kan*. To overcome these diseases a person should use *gu-gul* (gum-resin of *Commiphora mukul*), *brag-żun* (mineral pitch which comes out of the stones because of exposure to hot rays of the sun), *kyer-pa'i kha-ṇḍa* (solid extract from *Berberis aristata*) and honey. *'Bra-bu gsum* (three myrobalan fruits) mixed with honey also cures these ailments.

## Depletion Therapy

Depletion therapy is indicated for patients suffering from indigestion, obstinate urinary disorders including diabetes, internal abscess, gout, rheumatism, splenomegaly, diseases of the throat, head and heart, fever associated with diarrhoea, vomiting, heaviness of the body, nausea and obstruction in the passage of urine and stool. It is useful for a person who is physically strong, who is in his youth, and who indulges in fatty food. It is useful for persons having aggravated *mkhris-pa* and *bad-kan*, and during winter season.

Medicated recipes in the form of decoctions, powders, etc., which are stimulants of digestion and carminative are useful for this purpose. Physical exercise, fomentation therapy, hot bath, cauterisation therapy and blood-letting therapy cause depletion of the individual. Elimination therapies like vomiting therapy, purgation therapy and medicated enema therapy with the help of ununctuous decoctions, etc., cause depletion of the body.

If the depletion therapy is used in excess, then the person suffers from diminution of tissue elements, emaciation, giddiness, insomnia, loss of voice, lack of proper sense perception, loss of appetite, dryness of the mouth, pain in the calf region, thighs, sacro-iliac joint, head and heart, fever, delirium, vomiting sensation, and diseases caused by *rluṅ*.

Between an obese and emaciated persons, the latter is more amenable to therapies than the former.

## Line of Treatment of Aggravated Ñes-pas

The line of treatment of aggravated *rluṅ, mkhris-pa* and *bad-kan* with reference to diet, regimens, drugs, external therapies and internal therapies are as follows :

*Diet for Aggravated Rluṅ*

For the alleviation of aggravated *rluṅ*, sesame oil is the best which should be extensively used in food preparations and massage. Jaggery, wine, old ghee, mutton, meat of marmot, horse and donkey, garlic, onion, etc., are also useful in this condition.

*Regimens of Aggravated Rluṅ*

Staying in a dark house which is hot, and association with friends, pleasing talks, sleep in a warm bed and wearing of warm cloth are useful in alleviating *rluṅ*.

*Medicines for Aggravated Rluṅ*

Different rejuvenating recipes containing asafoetida, nutmeg, garlic, aconite, three myrobalan fruits and other ingredients having sweet, sour and saline tastes, and which are hot and unctuous are useful for the alleviation of *rluṅ*.

*External and Internal Therapies for Aggravated Rluṅ*

For the alleviation of *rluṅ*, massage with one year old ghee, fomentation therapy and oleating medicated enema prepared of old ghee are very useful.

### Diet for Aggravated Mkhris-pa

Fresh meat of bull and deer, cold water, cold tea, yoghurt, butter-milk, cooked dandelion, soup of the freshly harvested barley, gruel prepared of barley-flour, and cooling food and drinks are useful for the alleviation of *mkhris-pa*.

### Regimens for Aggravated Mkhris-pa

Exposure to cold wind, staying in the shade of trees, moving in parks, residing in a cold house located in the bank of a river or lake, abstinence from anger, leading a leisurely life, and use of perfumes are useful for the alleviation of *mkhris-pa*.

### Medicines for Aggravated Mkhris-pa

Decoctions of green herbs, camphor, sandal wood, cow's bile and ingredients which are sweet, bitter, astringent and cooling are useful for alleviation of *mkhris-pa*.

### External and Internal Therapies for Aggravated Mkhris-pa

Sprinkling of water with the instrument called water-wheel, blood-letting therapy, venesection and purgation therapy with the help of sweet drugs are useful for the alleviation of *mkhris-pa*.

### Diet for Aggravated Bad-kan

For the alleviation of aggravated *bad-kan*, fish, meat of sheep and wild yak, old grains, hot food, strong alcohol, hot water, water boiled by adding ginger, and ingredients which are light, ununctuous and hot are useful.

*Regimens for Aggravated Bad-kan*

Exposure to the heat of the sun and fire, wearing of warm cloth, residing in a hot place, exercise and remaining awake at night are useful for the alleviation of *bad-kan*.

*Medicines for Aggravated Bad-kan*

Decoctions added with saline and pungent ingredients, powder of pomegranate, and alkali preparations are useful for the alleviation of *bad-kan*.

*External and Internal Therapies for Aggravated Bad-kan*

Smoking and cauterisation therapies, and emetic therapy with sharp and ununctuous ingredients are useful for the alleviation of *bad-kan*.

Details of these and such other therapies, and lines of treatment are described in detail in the texts of Tibetan medicine.

# 13

# Important Medicinal Plants Used in Tibetan Medicine

As has been mentioned before, three categories of ingredients are used in Tibetan medicine, viz., (1) herbal products, (2) animal products, and (3) metals and minerals including costly stones. Of these, herbs are profusely used for medicinal purposes. Some of these herbs are available in Tibet and its adjoining areas like Laddakh, Sikkim, Bhutan and the high peaks of the Himalayas in Nepal and India. Some others, however, grow in Tropical areas which are imported. Because of their nonavailability, sometimes substitutes are used in their place in the recipes. Most of these herbs are identifiable and the teacher traditionally help the students to identify these herbs by taking them along to high peaks of mountains periodically. Identity of some others is, however, controversial, and different physicians use different plants in the same recipe.

Plants are treated as living beings. To uproot a plant is, therefore, considered unholy. But to save the human beings and animals from their miseries, the plant sacrifices itself like a saint sacrificing his own comforts of life for the welfare of others. The society respects the saints for their benevolent acts. Similarly, a plant is respected, and offered prayers before it is uprooted or cut for medicinal use. Religious rituals are performed before collecting them, and even after collecting them, rituals are performed to enhance their therapeutic efficacy.

Different parts of the plant are used in medicine because of therapeutic efficacy. Some plants, particularly the small herbs are used as a whole in medicine. But in the case of others, only a particular part of the plant is used. These parts become therapeutically potent in a particular season, and the physician is aware of it. Generally, physicians collect these plants and process themselves for the use of their patients. Large scale manufacture of medicines was generally not undertaken earlier. But in recent times such big manufacturing units are coming up to cater to the overgrowing demand of the patients. Of course, these large scale manufacturing units do observe these rules prescribed in the medical texts to some extent.

Some of the commonly used medicinal plants are described below.

## A-ru-ra (Terminalia chebula)

This is the most important medicinal plant, and its fruit is generally used in medicine. The right hand of the Medicine Buddha is adorned with the branch of this tree. There are many mythological stories about the origin of this medicinal plant. It is at the instruction of Lord Buddha, the seeds of this tree was planted in the mountain by the name *Spoṅs-ṅad-ldan (Gandha-mārdana?)* which is situated in the Eastern ghat range of the mountains in India. The root of this tree cures the diseases of bones; the trunk cures the diseases of muscle tissues; the branches of this tree cures the diseases of vessels and tendons; the bark cures the diseases of the skin; the leaf cures the diseases of *snod* (hollow visceras); the flower cures the diseases of sense organs, and the fruit cures the diseases of solid visceras like heart.

It is of five varieties as follows :

(1)   *Rnam-gyal* (the victorious one);
(2)   *'Jigs-med* (the fearless one);
(3)   *Bdud-rtsi* (the one like ambrosia);
(4)   *'Phel-byed* (the growth promoting one); and
(5)   *Skem-pa* (the emaciated one).

At present only a few of these varieties could be identified. This tree is endowed with all the six tastes, eight *nus-pas* (potencies), three *żu-rjes* (the taste that emerges after digestion) and seventeen types of *yon-tan* (attributes).

It is used in number of recipes of Tibetan medicine. It promotes longevity, and stimulates the power of digestion. It is carminative and wholesome for the body. Because of its efficacy to alleviate all the three *ñes-pas*, viz., *rluṅ, mkhris-pa* and *bad-kan*, it cures all the four hundred and four diseases.

## Ba-ru-ra (Terminalia belerica)

Like *a-ru-ra*, this *ba-ru-ra* is a big tree. It alleviates *bad-kan* and *mkhris-pa*. It cures diseases caused by the vitiation of lymph.

## Skyu-ru-ra (Emblica officinalis)

It is a medium-size tree. Its fruit cures diseases caused by *bad-kan* and *mkhris-pa*. It corrects the vitiation of blood.

## Na-le-sam (Piper nigrum)

It alleviates *bad-kan* and cures diseases caused by cold.

## Pi-pi-liṅ (Piper longum)

Long pepper cures all the diseases caused by cold without exception.

## Sman-sgas (Zingiber officinalis)

The freshly harvested and the dried rhizomes of this plant are extensively used in medicine to stimulate the power of digestion. It alleviates *bad-kan* and *rluṅ*. It liquefies the thickened blood.

## Ga-bur (Cinnamomum camphora)

The resin of this tree is used in medicine. It is also extracted from the leaves and barks of this tree by the process of distillation and sublimation. It cures acute fever afflicting the head (meningitis). It also cures chronic and persistent fever.

## Tsan-dan dkar-po (Santalum album)

The white variety of sandal-wood cures diseases of the head and heart. It also cures fever associated with diarrhoea.

## Tsan-dan dmar-po (Pterocarpus santalum)

The red variety of sandal-wood cures fevers caused by the vitiation of blood.

## Gu-gul (Commiphora mukul)

The gum-resin of this tree is used in medicine. It cures ailments caused by the seizures of evil spirits. It also cures obstinate types of ulcer, and acute pain.

## Sug-smel (Elettaria cardamomum)

Fruits and seeds are used in medicine. It cures kidney diseases, and all diseases caused by cold.

## *Ka-ko-la (Amomum subulatum)*

Fruits and seeds of this plant are used in medicine. It cures diseases of stomach and spleen caused by their affliction with cold.

## *Gur-gum (Crocus sativus)*

It is of different types, one is cultivated in Kashmir, the other is brought from Nepal, and the third type is found in Tibet. The saffron of Kashmir is considered to be the best, and it is the androcum in the flowers of this plant which is used in recipes. Because of the high cost involved, and less availability, the androcum of another plant called *Carthamus tinctorius* is used in its place in ordinary recipes.

It cures liver-disorders and stops bleeding.

## *Cu-gaṅ (Bambusa bambos)*

It is an exudate available in old bamboos and popularly known as bamboo-manna. It is an excellent remedy for all types of lungs-diseases. It also cures fever and different types of ulcer.

## *Tig-ta (Swertia chirata)*

This bitter drug cures all types of fever caused by the aggravation of *mkhris-pa*.

## *Sñiṅ-źo-sa (Spondias axillaris)*

There are three types of *źo-sa*, viz., (1) *sñiṅ-źo-sa* which cures heart diseases, (2) *mkhal-ma źo-sa* which cures kidney diseases, and (3) *Gla-gar zo-sa* which cures spleen diseases.

## Hoṅ-len (Picrorhiza kurroa)

The rhizome of this plant is used in medicine. It is very bitter in taste. It cures fever associated with diarrhoea. It also cures different types of fever caused by the affliction of solid visceras.

## Star-bu (Garcinia pedunculata)

It produces drying effect on the lungs, and stops haemoptysis. It also stops excessive expectoration from *bad-kan*.

## Dzā-ti (Myristica fragrance)

Nut-meg alleviates *rluṅ*, and cures all types of heart diseases.

## Dug-mo ñuṅ (Holarrhena antidysenterica)

It alleviates *mkhris-pa*, and cures fever associated with diarrhoea.

## Thal-ka rdo-rje (Cassia tora)

It cures skin diseases and diseases of the lymph.

## Gser gyi me-tog (Momordica charantia)

It cures diseases of hollow visceras. It also cures fevers caused by the aggravation of *mkhris-pa*.

## La-la-phud (Trachyspermum ammi)

It cures stomach disorders, and diseases caused by cold.

## Na-ga ge-sar (Mesua ferrea)

It cures diseases of lungs, liver and heart.

## Byi-taṅ-ga (Embelia ribes)

It improves the power of digestion, and cures parasitic infestations.

## Ma-nu (Inula helenium)

It cures fever caused by the aggravation of *rluṅ* and vitiation of blood.

## 'Jam-'bras (Syzygium cumini)

It cures diseases of kidneys.

## Boṅ-ṅa (dkar-po) (Aconitum heterophyllum)

It is of three varieties, viz., white, red and yellow. The white variety cures infectious fever, poisoning and fever caused by *mkhris-pa*. The red and yellow varieties cure ailments caused by meat-poisoning and aconite poisoning.

## Śiṅ-mṅar (Glycyrrhiza glabra)

Liquorice cures diseases of the lungs, and cleanses the channels of circulation.

## Pri-ya-ṅgu (Aglaia roxburghiana)

It cures fever caused by the affliction of stomach and liver.

### Par-pa-ṭa (Fumaria parviflora)

It cures infectious fever, and fever caused by poisoning.

### Gze-ma (Tribulus terrestris)

Its seeds are used for curing dysuria, gout and kidney-diseases.

### Ru-rta (Saussurea lappa)

The root of this plant is used in medicine. It cures *rluṅ* and vitiated blood. It also cures flatulence, diseases of lungs, and obstruction in the throat. It prevents decaying of muscle tissue.

### Spos-dkar (Shorea robusta)

The gum exudate of this tree is used in medicine. It purifies and dries up lymph.

### U' su (Coriandrum sativum)

Coriander cures stomach-diseases caused by the aggravation of *bad-kan*, and fever.

### Li-śi (Syzygium aromaticum)

Cloves alleviate cold type of *rluṅ*. It cures diseases caused by the affliction of the channels carrying vital air.

### Se-'bru (Punica granatum)

Pomegranate cures all the diseases of the stomach. It stimulates the gastric fire. It also cures all the diseases caused by *bad-kan* and cold.

The medicinal plants described above with reference to their important therapeutic properties, are the frequently used ones. There are several others having important therapeutic effects. Though rarely used some of these hold high promise for future research work because these are efficacious in curing various obstinate and otherwise incurable diseases.

# 14

# Popular Recipes Used for Treatment of Common Diseases

Therapeutic properties of drugs of plant and animal origin, metals, minerals, gems and costly stones are described in detail in the works of Tibetan medicine. Very often these drugs as such (single drugs) are used by the physicians for the treatment of their patients. Some of these drugs in their natural form are toxic. Even if these are detoxified by processing them through prescribed methods, some of them are so potent that in certain circumstances, these are likely to produce some adverse reactions in the body of the patient. Therefore, these are administered along with other drugs which counteract these adverse effects. Some of these are not of good taste. To neutralise their bad taste, some other palatable drugs are added. These natural products have their limitations in their therapeutic efficacy. At times, these are to be administered in a big dose to produce the desired results. It may become difficult for some patients to take them in such a big dose. To make such drugs more potent to be effective only in a small dose, some other drugs having synergistic action are added. Diseases are of different types, and each one of these diseases has many varieties. It is therefore, difficult for the physician to maintain a huge drug store to cater to the requirements of different types of patients. Therefore, to the original one, some other drugs are added to make the therapy multi-dimensional and multifaceted. Keeping the above points in view, different recipes containing several drugs are formulated and used in therapeutics by the Tibetan physician.

In addition, these recipes of compound drugs are to be made easily administrable, digestible, assimilable, tolerable and preservable for which different pharmaceutical processes are adopted by the physician and manufacturer. For these single drugs and compound formulations, the pharmaceutical preparations are made of the following categories :

(1)   *Phye-ma* or powders;
(2)   *Ril-bu* or pills;
(3)   *Thaṅ* or decoctions;
(4)   *Lde-gu* or linctus;
(5)   *Sman-mar* or medicated ghee and oil;
(6)   *Thal-sman* or calcined preparations of metals and minerals including gems and costly stones;
(7)   *Khaṇd(r)a* or semi-solid water extract prepared by concentrating decoctions;
(8)   *Sman-chaṅ* or medicated wines; and
(9)   *Rin-chen* or recipes containing gems and costly stones.

Different processes involved in the preparation of these various categories of recipes are elaborated in Tibetan medical works.

## Purification of Toxic Ingredients

Some drugs, in their natural form are toxic to the human body. These are made non-toxic before being administered in the form of either single drugs or compound formulations. This is called the process of purification. Apart from removing physical and chemical impurities, at times, this process involves boiling and triturating with the juice or decoction of plants, and urine, bile, etc., of animals to make a new organic compound which not only makes the drug non-toxic, but also becomes easily assimilable. The drug, thus becomes therapeutically more effective. For example, aconite is often used in the recipes of the formulations of Tibetan medicine. In raw form, it is toxic because of its cardiac-depressant property. Before use, it is cut into small pieces, and boiled with cow's urine or milk by which it becomes cardiac stimulant.

## Naming a Recipe

Most of these compound formulations have a name of title by which these are described in the medical texts and prescribed by the physicians. These names or titles of compound formulations are based on the following :

(1) The recipe, at times, is named after the important ingredient in it;

(2) Sometime the recipe is named after the name of the original propounder of the formulation;

(3) The recipe, at times, is named on the basis of the therapeutic effect of the recipe; and

(4) At times, the recipe is named after the first ingredient appearing in the formulation which is suffixed by the total number of ingredients.

Apart from ingredients composing the recipe, the quantity of each ingredient, the part of the plant to be used, the method to be followed for processing the recipe, the vehicles to be used along with the recipe and its therapeutic effects are described while presenting such a formulation. Since these formulations are generally memorised by the physician, the description is often in brief, and in obvious cases description of some of these topics is omitted. Each student of Tibetan medicine has to memorise these, at least some of the important recipes, and trained practically to prepare them in front of the teacher.

Some of the popular recipes generally used for the treatment of common ailments are described below by way of illustration.

## Bsam-'phel Nor-bu

| | Ingredients | Parts Used | Quantity |
|---|---|---|---|
| (1) | *Cu-gaṅ* (Bamboo-salt) | Exudate | 1 Gm. |
| (2) | *Gur-gum* (Saffron) | Androcium | 3.5 Gm. |
| (3) | *Li-śi* (Clove) | Fruit | 3.5 Gm. |
| (4) | *Dzā-ti* (Nut-meg) | Fruit | 6 Gm. |
| (5) | *Sug-smel* (Small Cardamom) | Seed | 3.5 Gm. |
| (6) | *Ka-ko-la* (Big Cardamom) | Seed | 1 Gm. |
| (7) | *Tsan-dan Dkar-po* (White Sandal-wood) | Heart wood | 3 Gm. |
| (8) | *Tsan-dan Dmar-po* (Red Sandal-wood) | Heart wood | 40 Gm. |
| (9) | *A-gar Nag-po* (*Aquilaria agallocha*) | Heart wood | 3 Gm. |
| (10) | *Gla-rtsi* (Musk) | Animal product (exudate) | 3 Gm. |
| (11) | *Ghi-vaṅ* (Solidified Cattle-bile) | Animal product | 5 Gm. |
| (12) | *Mu-tig* (Pearl) | Animal product | 10 Gm. |
| (13) | *Bśe-ru* (Rhinoceros) | Animal product (horn) | 5 Gm. |

*contd...*

| Ingredients | Parts Used | Quantity |
| --- | --- | --- |
| (14) *A-ru-ra (Terminalia chebula)* | Fruit-pulp | 3.5 Gm. |
| (15) *Ba-ru-ra (Terminalia belerica)* | Fruit-pulp | 3.5 Gm. |
| (16) *Skyu-ru-ra (Emblica officinalis)* | Fruit-pulp | 5 Gm. |
| (17) *Zi-ra Dkar-po* (White Cumin seed) | Seed | 3.5 Gm. |
| (18) *Zi-ra Nag-po* (Black Cumin seed) | Seed | 3.5 Gm. |
| (19) *Pi-pi-liṅ* (Long pepper) | Fruit | 3.5 Gm. |
| (20) *Sga-dmar* (Ginger) | Rhizome | 3.5 Gm. |
| (21) *Śiṅ-tshwa* (Cinnamon) | Bark | 2.5 Gm. |
| (22) *Spos-dkar (Shorea robusta)* | Exudate | 4 Gm. |
| (23) *Thal-ka rdor-rdze (Cassia tora)* | Seed | 4 Gm. |
| (24) *So-ma ra-dza (Psoralea corylifolia)* | Seed | 4 Gm. |
| (25) *Ma-nu (Inula racemosa)* | Root | 2 Gm. |
| (26) *Ru-rta (Saussurea lappa)* | Root | 2 Gm. |
| (27) *Śiṅ-mṅar (Glycyrrhiza glabra)* | Stem | 4 Gm. |
| (28) *Sa-'dzin* | Plant | 4 Gm. |
| (29) *Gser-bye* | Fruit | 3.5 Gm. |
| (30) *Sdig-pa* (An insect) | Animal | 3.5 Gm. |

## Lat-thabs (Method of Preparation)

This recipe is generally prepared in the form of pills. Item no. 12, i.e. *mu-tig* or pearl is to be reduced to powder form according to the prescribed procedure. Item no. 30 is dried well before pounding. All the ingredients, except item nos. 10 & 11 (musk and cattle bile) are to be made powder separately, and thereafter, mixed together. To this powder, item nos. 10 & 11 should be added. By adding water, all these ingredients are to be triturated well and made to a paste. From out of this paste, pills of 250 mg. each, should be prepared and dried in the shade. These pills should be rapped with pieces or silken cloth and stored in a clean and dry glass bottle.

## Nus pa (Therapeutic Indications)

It is an excellent recipe for the promotion of immunitary system. It cures cancer, gout, rheumatic, rheumatoid and osteo-arthritis, spondylitis, osteoporosis, obstinate skin-diseases including leprosy and diseases of kidneys.

## Thun (Dosage)

One or two pills to be taken in the morning.

## Sman-rta (Vehicles)

These pills become very effective when given along with warm milk or warm water.

To make these pills therapeutically more potent to cure some of the obstinate and otherwise incurable diseases, special religious rituals are performed before giving to the patients.

## A-ru Bdun-pa

| Ingredients | Parts used | Quantity |
|---|---|---|
| (1) *A-ru-ra* (*Terminalia chebula*) | Fruit pulp | 100 Gm. |
| (2) *Cu-gan* (Bamboo-salt) | Exudate | 50 Gm. |
| (3) *Sin-mnar* (*Glycyrrhiza glabra*) | Stem | 50 Gm. |
| (4) *Pan-rgyan dkar-po* | Plant | 50 Gm. |
| (5) *Sra-lo* | Plant | 50 Gm. |
| (6) *Sug-smel* (Small Cardamom) | Seed | 50 Gm. |
| (7) *Li-si* (Clove) | Fruit | 50 Gm. |

## Las-thab (Method of Preparation)

This recipe is generally used in pill form. All the ingredients are made to powder form separately and then mixed together. By adding water, this is triturated and made to a paste. From out of this paste, pills of 250 mg. each, are prepared. These are dried and kept in a glass bottle.

## Nus-pa (Therapeutic Indications)

These pills are useful for curing all the seven types of throat diseases including hoarseness of the voice.

## Thun (Dosage)

Two pills three times per day, i.e. morning, noon and evening.

## Sman-rta (Vehicle)

Hot water after making slightly cool.

## Skyer-sun Brgyad-pa

| Ingredients | Part Used | Quantity |
|---|---|---|
| (1) Skyer-śun (*Berberis aristata*) | Stem bark | 100 Gm. |
| (2) Pi-pi-liṅ (Long pepper) | Fruit | 40 Gm. |
| (3) Skyu-ru-ra (*Emblica officinalis*) | Fruit pulp | 25 Gm. |
| (4) Śiṅ-mṅar (*Glycyrrhiza glabra*) | Stem | 40 Gm. |
| (5) Gla-rtsi (Musk) | Animal product | 40 Gm. |
| (6) Kha-che Gur-gum (Saffron) | Androceum | 25 Gm. |
| (7) Dom-mkhris (Bear-bile) | Animal product | 75 Gm. |
| (8) Rgya-snag | Mineral | 75 Gm. |

## Las-thab (Method of Preparation)

The recipe is generally used in the form of powder. In the beginning, powders of item nos. 1 to 4, 6 and 8 should be prepared separately. To this, the powders of the item nos. 5 and 6 should be added and mixed well. This powder should be stored in an airtight and clean glass bottle.

## Nus-pa (Therapeutic Indications)

This is useful for dysuria and obstinate urinary disorders.

## Thun (Dosage)

Half gram of this powder should be given to the patient twice daily, both morning and evening.

## Sman-rta (Vehicle)

Hot water.

### Ga-bur Bcu-bźi

| Ingredients | Part Used | Quantity |
|---|---|---|
| (1) *Ga-bur* (Camphor) | Exudate | 100 Gm. |
| (2) *Dzā-ti* (Nutmeg) | Fruit | 25 Gm. |
| (3) *Li-śi* (Clove) | Fruit | 25 Gm. |
| (4) *Cu-gań* (Bamboo-salt) | Exudate | 25 Gm. |
| (5) *Gur-gum* (Saffron) | Androceum | 25 Gm. |
| (6) *Sug-smel* (Small Cardamom) | Seed | 25 Gm. |
| (7) *Ka-ko-la* (Big Cardamom) | Seed | 25 Gm. |
| (8) *Tsan-dan Dkar-po* | Heart wood | 25 Gm. |
| (9) *Bśe-ru* (Rhinoceros) | Horn | 15 Gm. |
| (10) *Utpal* (Lotus) | Flower | 25 Gm. |
| (11) *A-gar* (*Aquilaria agallocha*) | Heart wood | 25 Gm. |
| (12) *Gla-rtsi* (Musk) | Animal product | 10 Gm. |
| (13) *Tig-ta* (*Swertia chirata*) | Plant | 25 Gm. |
| (14) *Li-ga-dur* | Root | 15 Gm. |

## Las-thabs (Method of Preparation)

This recipe is generally used in the form of pills. Powder of all ingredients, except item nos. 1 and 12, should be mixed well and triturated by adding small quantity of sugar and water. After it is reduced to a fine paste form, item nos. 1 and 12 should be added further triturated. From out of this fine paste, pills of 250 mg. each should be prepared and dried in the shade. These pills should be stored in a clean and dry glass bottle, and properly corked.

## Nus-pa (Therapeutic Indications)

It is useful in all types of fever including malaria and meningitis, delirium, fainting and malaise.

## Thus (Dosage)

Two pills should be taken twice daily, once at the noon time and once at night.

## Sman-rta (Vehicle)

Hot water after it is slightly cooled.

### Tig-ta Brgyad-pa

| Ingredients | Part Used | Quantity |
| --- | --- | --- |
| (1) *Tig-ta* (*Swertia chirata*) | Whole plant | 100 Gm. |
| (2) *Gser-me* (*Momordica charantia*) | Fruit | 80 Gm. |
| (3) *Boṅ-dkar* (*Aconitum heterophylum*) | Root | 80 Gm. |
| (4) *Ru-rta* (*Saussurea lappa*) | Root | 80 Gm. |
| (5) *Rtsa-mkhris* | Whole plant | 80 Gm. |

*contd...*

| Ingredients | Part Used | Quantity |
|---|---|---|
| (6) *Hoṅ-len* (*Picrorhiza kurroa*) | Rhizome | 50 Gm. |
| (7) *Pa-pa-ṭa* (*Fumaria parviflora*) | Whole plant | 40 Gm. |
| (8) *Skyer-śun* (*Berberis aristata*) | Stem | 70 Gm. |

## Las-thabs (Method of Preparation)

This recipe is generally used in the form of pills. All these ingredients are to be made to powders separately, and mixed well. To make the recipe more potent, 80 Gms. of *doms-mkhris* (bear bile) may be added. By adding water, the mixture should be triturated well to make it a fine paste. From out of this, pills of 250 mg. each, should be prepared and dried. These pills are to be stored in a dry and clean glass bottle.

## Nus-pa (Therapeutic Indications)

Bilious fever, jaundice and different types of hepatitis.

## Thun (Dosage)

Two pills twice daily, one during mid-day and once during mid-night.

## Sman-rta (Vehicle)

Boiled water after completely cooled.

## Tsan-dan Bco-brgyad

| Ingredients | Part Used | Quantity |
| --- | --- | --- |
| (1) *Tsan-dan* (Sandal-wood) | Heart wood | 15 Gm. |
| (2) *Ghi-vam* (Cattle bile) | Animal product | 5 Gm. |
| (3) *Dzā-ti* (Nut-meg) | Fruit | 2.5 Gm. |
| (4) *Li-si* (Clove) | Fruit | 2.5 Gm. |
| (5) *Cu-gaṅ* (Bamboo-salt) | Exudate | 2.5 Gm. |
| (6) *Gur-gum* (Safforn) | Androceum | 2.5 Gm. |
| (7) *Sug-smel* (Small Cardamom) | Seed | 2.5 Gm. |
| (8) *Ka-ko-la* (Big Cardamom) | Seed | 2.5 Gm. |
| (9) *A-ru-ra* (*Terminalia chebula*) | Fruit pulp | 5 Gm. |
| (10) *Sum-cu-tig* | Whole plant | 5 Gm. |
| (11) *Ru-rta* (*Saussurea lappa*) | Root | 5 Gm. |
| (12) *Rgya-skyegs* (Lac) | Exudate | 5 Gm. |
| (13) *Pri-yaṅ-ku* | Flower | 5 Gm. |
| (14) *Hoṅ-len* (*Picrorhiza kurroa*) | Rhizome | 5 Gm. |
| (15) *Re-skon* | Whole plant | 5 Gm. |
| (16) *Ba-sa-ka* | Whole plant | 5 Gm. |
| (17) *Btsod* (*Rubia cordifolia*) | Stem | 5 Gm. |
| (18) *'Bri-mog* | Root | 5 Gm. |

## Las-thabs (Method of Preparation)

This recipe is generally prepared in the form of powder. All the ingredients, except item no. 2, are made to powders separately, and then mixed together. Thereafter, item no. 2 is made to powder, added to the recipe and mixed well. This is then stored in a clean and dry glass jar.

## Nus-pa (Therapeutic Indications)

This recipe is useful in diarrhoea, vomiting, pain in the chest and back, heart diseases, cramps, headache, eye diseases, liver disorders, ulcer in the stomach, and colitis.

## Thun (Dosage)

500 mg. twice daily in empty stomach.

## Sman-rta (Vehicle)

Hot water after slightly cooled.

The recipes described above are only by the way of illustration. Several other recipes are described in Tibetan Medical texts and used by Tibetan physicians for curing common ailments, and also diseases which are considered to be serious and otherwise incurable. These recipes have stood the test of time, and used by the suffering humanity for thousands of years. There are, of course controversies about the identification of some of these ingredients, and there are variations in the composition, etc., of these recipes. Such controversies and variations are natural because of temporal factor and lack of communication in the ancient and medieval period.

Tibetan tradition and culture were often painted as mysterious. Religious and philosophical studies apart, very little attention has been paid towards the studies of its secular and scientific traditions. More recently, scientists are evincing keen interest in the Medical Science of Tibet. Several drugs used in this system are botanically identified. Clinical and scientific studies of these recipes and single drugs under controlled conditions have not been seriously attempted so far. Recipes apart, the fundamental principles, if studied properly and applied for the preservation and promotion of positive health, and prevention as well as cure of diseases, will be a great boon to mitigate the ailments, physical, mental and spiritual, suffering of the humanity.

## 15

# Physician and Medical Practice

The physician of Traditional Tibetan medicine is an embodiment of all the physical, mental, moral and spiritual virtues. According to Tibetan tradition, the knowledge (*rig-gnas*), both religious and secular, are of ten categories. The major five categories (*che-ba lṅa*) are as follows :

(1) *Bzo-rig-pa* or technology, etc.;
(2) *Gso-ba rig-pa* or medicine;
(3) *Sgra'i rig-pa* or grammar;
(4) *Tshad-ma rig-pa* or logic; and
(5) *Naṅ-don rig-pa.*

The remaining minor five categories (*Chun-ba lṅa*) are as follows :

(6) *Sñan-daṅs* or poetics;
(7) *Sdeb-sbyor* or metrics;
(8) *Mṅon-brjod* or lexicon;
(9) *Zlos-gar* or dramatics; and
(10) *Rtsis* or astrology.

The physician should be prudent scholar of his own branch of knowledge, i.e. Gso-ba rig-pa or the science and art of medicine. In addition, he should be well versed with the remaining branches of knowledge. He should never commit ten types of sins through his body, mind and speech.

The primary objectives of entering into medical profession are as follows :

(1) To maintain positive health, and prevent as well as cure diseases;

(2) To promote longevity by which a person can adequately perform his religious duties, earn his livelihood, satisfy sensual desires and attain *nirvāṇa* or salvation;

(3) To make living creatures free from miseries; and

(4) To attain excellence and respect from others.

In view of the respect shown by the society to the medical profession, very often unqualified and inexperienced persons enter into the profession for livelihood and endanger the life of the patient. Such quacks are to be identified and their practice of medicine has to be discouraged by the ruler of land with strong hand.

Wisdom, purity of mind, keeping a promise, dexterity in different fields of knowledge, expertise in medical profession and scholarship in religious affairs—these are the natural dispositions of a physician. He possesses expansive as well as determinative wisdom for subtle analysis of mundane and transcendental phenomena.

Because of the purity of mind, the physician gets endowed with the spirit of Lord Buddha (*chub-sems*) which is free from all the sins and defilements, and enters into *sbyor-ba* state. He visualises miseries of his patients and gets involved in beneficial activities for all living being with love. To him, pleasure and pain, and friendship and enmity become equal. Because of this state of mind, he practises the following four principles of medical profession :

(1) *Sñiṅ-rje* or compassion for the suffering humanity;

(2) *Byam-pa* or friendship with patients to treat them as his own relatives;

(3) *Dga'-ba* or happiness in attempting treatment of the curable patients; and

(4) *Btan-snoms* or desertation of the incurable patients.

He is committed to the vow of practising the incantation of *Sman-lha* (Medicine Buddha) as follows :

"OM NA MO BHA GA WA TE BHAI SA DZYE GU RU
   BAI DU RYA
PRA BHA RA DZA YA TA THA GA TA YA A RHA TE
   SA MYA KSAM BU
DDHA YA, TA DYA THA, OM BHAI SA DZYE BHAI
   SA DZYE,
MA HA BHAI SA DZYE, BHAI SA DZYA RA DZA YA?
SA MU DGA TE SWA HA.

Continuous recitation of this incantation of Medicine Buddha bestows blessings on himself, on his patients and on his medicaments.

A physician is defined as a person who treats diseases, who prescribes medicines for the benefit of the body, who bravely handles a patient after the latter's recovery from disease, and who protects a patient like his father. Apart from his general duties described above, the duties to be performed by him through his body, mind and speech are described in great detail in Tibetan texts.

Practice of medical profession endows a physician with two types of benefits, viz., temporary and eternal. The temporary benefits accrue to the physician during his life time. He gets endowed with strength, pleasure of life and happiness. As eternal benefit, he becomes free from illusion and worldly desires. After death he enters into the abode of Lord Buddha, the Supreme Healer and Teacher.

# Index

(Medicinal Ingredients : Arranged in
Roman Alphabetical Order)